LIFE AFTER LIMB LOSS

A Guide for New Amputees and Their Families

*To Nina,
Hope this book is helpful to your clients & peers!
Best
Julie Gross PT*

JULIE GROSS, P.T.

Copyright © 2018 Julie Gross
All rights reserved.

ISBN: 978-0-9979486-3-9

DISCLAIMER

The information in this book is intended for educational and informational purposes. It is not meant to and should not be used to diagnose or substitute for medical treatment. You should discuss any new exercises, medications, or other treatments with your doctor before trying them. For diagnosis and treatment of a medical problem you should see your physician. The publisher and author are not responsible for any specific health needs that may require medical supervision and are not liable for negative consequences from actions resulting from reading or following the information in this book. Any links to outside resources are not under the control of the publisher or author and may change at any time.

The stories in this book are from real people who have consented to share their stories, and the experiences of the author. The do not represent any suggestions on appropriate medical care. Each person is different, and you should consult a medical professional before you undertake any new courses of care.

In memory of David D. Kilmer, MD
My mentor, inspiration, and friend.

Contents

Introduction	1
Part I: Amputations	**3**
Chapter 1: Reasons for Amputations	5
Chapter 2: Types of Amputations	15
Chapter 3: Personal Stories	19
Part II: Recovery Phases after an Amputation	**37**
Chapter 4: Reacting to the News	39
Chapter 5: Family Reactions	49
Part III: Post-Operative Phase	**53**
Chapter 6: The Team	55
Chapter 7: Hospital to Home	57
Chapter 8: Phantom Limb Sensation and Phantom Limb	61
Chapter 9: Exercises	63
Chapter 10: Prosthetic Fitting	73
Part IV: Moving Forward/Acceptance	**89**
Chapter 11: Physical needs	91
Chapter 12: Emotional needs	95
Chapter 13: Advice from Our Amputees	97
Conclusion	105
Acknowledgements	107

Introduction

No one ever wishes to lose a limb. And there are many different reasons lower limb loss occurs. This book will hopefully challenge you to rethink your idea of what an amputation means.

Amputation is still often viewed as a failure of treatment. This perception of failed treatment needs to change. Whatever the reason for performing an extremity amputation, it is a treatment of choice and is always performed as a life-saving procedure. Patients and family members must be aware of their options and have realistic expectations of surgical outcomes to make informed decisions regarding amputation. For some, it is an easy decision, while for others it is a very difficult choice.

The purpose of this book is twofold. First, I hope this book can be a guide for those new to amputation—helping all new amputees and their families understand the common, characteristic steps for adjusting to their new life. Second, and more important, I hope this book provides others with the opportunity to meet "everyday" people with lower limb loss who have succeeded in living full, meaningful lives. These amputees are willing to share their personal stories of new and different lives following limb loss. All of the featured stories have common threads of inner strength, determination, faith, and gratitude.

The stories shared here are from a very diverse group of patients that I have worked with and befriended after years of following them through their individual transitions. I am excited to share their journeys and to help assist others through this book.

This book is written for the everyday patient that suffered the progression of their disease, was born with missing limb(s), or had a traumatic accident.

How did I get here? In high school, I recognized that my career passion was healthcare and more specifically the field of physical therapy. I soon recognized my love and talent as a rehabilitation physical therapist, which led me to become a specialist in the area of lower limb loss. I have been a clinical instructor at the University of Missouri, and have provided educational and clinical training to physical therapy interns, residents, and physicians for the past 30 years. During my transition from Missouri to California, I continued the pursuit of my expertise in lower limb rehabilitation and provided presentations at symposiums and local hospitals in the Sacramento/Bay Area in California. I've had the pleasure of working with world renowned physical therapy clinicians and prosthetists. I am blessed to be considered the Northern Californian region's Prosthetic Physical Therapy Specialist, which offers me the opportunity to receive referral clients from all over Northern California.

My experiences have led me to identify patterns in both clients who succeed in their rehabilitation and those who struggle to regain their former lives. I believe that every person is an individual with unique experiences, which shapes our ability to adjust and react to changes. In cases involving amputation, some clients have smoother transitions and understanding including the ability to learn from their successes. The patterns associated with these cases may help others during their individual rehabilitation and initial challenges after an amputation.

PART 1

Amputations

CHAPTER 1

Reasons for Amputations

There are many reasons and sometimes complicating factors for why someone may have an amputation. Sometimes it is a choice that is made after several years of input from friends, family, and doctors. Other times, the decision is made quickly in the hospital or emergency room with no real alternatives. In this chapter, you will learn some of the more common causes of amputation.

Let's begin with the possible medical reasons for amputation. There is a misperception that the number one reason for amputation is war-related injuries. With the onset of the Iraqi and Afghanistan Wars, and recent worldwide terrorist bombings, survivor stories are frequently in the forefront of all media outlets. The media is a great source for inspirational, survival accounts. Survivors of these horrific events bravely share their amazing stories, which help motivate us all to keep working toward achieving our goals. Often these portrayals, however, highlight survivors with lower limb loss.

These are truly heroic stories. The majority of limb loss today though is due to health issues and disease. Luckily, amputation is rarely due to wars and bombs. The most common causes of lower limb amputations are due to progressive diseases. The most common diseases being: vascular disease, including diabetes and peripheral arterial disease (54%), trauma (45%), and cancer (less than 2%). These diseases and their increased potential for amputation are discussed in upcoming chapters. While smoking is not a disease, the impact of smoking on peripheral vascular disease will also be discussed.

Below is an overview of statistics regarding amputation from Advanced Amputee Solutions (a veteran-owned medical device company, specializing in the development of amputee specific devices) updated in 2012:

- *Diabetes affects 25.8 million people, 8.3% of the U.S. population. About 1.9 million people aged 20 years or older were newly diagnosed with diabetes in 2010 in the United States.*
- *Diabetes rates vary by race, ethnicity, and age; with African-Americans & Native Americans at the top of the list.*
- *The number of amputations caused by diabetes increased by 24% from 1988 to 2009.*
- *Below-knee amputations are the most common amputations, representing 71% of dysvascular amputations; there is a 47% expected increase in below knee amputations from 1995-2020.*
- *The Amputee Coalition of America estimates that there are 185,000 new lower extremity amputations each year just within the United States and an estimated population of two million American amputees.*
- *It is projected that the amputee population will more than double by the year 2050 to 3.6 million.*
- *The estimated cost to American private & public insurance agencies is $12 billion annually.*
- *As of Sept. 1, 2010, there have been 1,621 new U.S. amputee "Wounded Warriors" as a result of Operation Iraqi Freedom, Operation Enduring Freedom, and Operation New Dawn.*
- *There are more than 1 million annual limb amputations globally ——one every 30 seconds——is even more troubling, particularly since the International Diabetes Federation (IDF) predicts that current global prevalence of diabetes will burgeon from 285 million to reach 435 million by 2030.*

- *Estimates suggest that more than 6% of the population aged 20–79 years in EU countries, or 33 million people, have diabetes in 2010.*

Vascular disease, which includes diabetes, blood clots (thrombosis), and atherosclerosis is the leading cause of amputation. The statistics above demonstrate the risks these diseases create, which can lead to an amputation.

Below are some of the most common causes of amputation

Peripheral Vascular Disease

Peripheral vascular disease (PVD) is a blood circulation disorder where the blood vessels become narrowed and blood flow decreases, becomes blocked, or may spasm. This can happen in your arteries or veins. Loss of circulation is the major cause of amputations.

Peripheral Vascular Disease symptoms typically cause pain and fatigue, often in your legs, and especially during exercise; the pain usually improves with rest. The medical term for these symptoms is claudication or intermittent claudication.

The medical terminology can sometimes be confusing, but in general, Peripheral Vascular Disease is also called the following:

- arteriosclerosis obliterans
- arterial insufficiency of the legs
- claudication
- intermittent claudication

Simply put, PVD is another cause of severe loss of circulation to your limbs, which as it progresses, may lead to limb amputation. As a reminder, amputation due to PVD is a lifesaving measure and can result in less pain and a more functional life.

Diabetes

Diabetes is a type of Peripheral Vascular Disease. It is a progressive disease, which can set the stage for amputations. As the disease progresses, the loss of circulation and blood flow to the legs can cause numbness in the feet. This numbness and loss of sensation is called diabetic neuropathy and is permanent nerve damage. Diabetic neuropathies cause someone to become less aware or unaware altogether of any injuries and ulcers that develop on their feet. These ulcers may fail to heal, which can in turn lead to serious infections. The only treatment option at this last stage is amputation.

Arteriosclerosis and Blood Clots (Thrombosis)

Arteriosclerosis and blood clots are also a form of Peripheral Vascular Disease. These diseases, like diabetes, are progressive and may lead to limb loss, particularly amputation of lower legs. With arteriosclerosis, or "hardening of the arteries," plaques build up in a vessel and limit the flow of blood and oxygen to your organs and limbs. As plaque growth progresses, blood clots may develop and completely block the artery. This can lead to organ damage and loss of fingers, toes, or limbs if left untreated.

Blood clots form when there is damage to the lining of a blood vessel. Thrombosis is the medical term for a blood clot formation inside a blood vessel, which obstructs the flow of blood through the circulatory system. Thrombosis may occur in the veins or the arteries. If the blood clot or a piece of the clot breaks free and travels through the body, it is called an embolus. An embolus traveling through your arteries can become stuck and restrict blood flow. Arterial blood clots affect the arms, legs, and feet. An arterial embolus can lead to complete blockage of blood supply to an extremity, and this condition is called acute limb ischemia. If there is a complete blockage, amputation of the limb may be medically necessary.

Peripheral Artery Disease

Peripheral arterial disease (PAD) develops only in the arteries, which carry oxygen-rich blood away from the heart. According to the CDC, approximately 12-20% of people over age 60 develop PAD, about 8.5 million people in the United States. PAD is the most common form of PVD so the terms are often used to mean the same condition.

Smoking

The leading cause of peripheral vascular disease is smoking. The general public associates smoking with lung cancer and heart diseases such as heart attacks & strokes. However, vascular disease is the second leading cause of amputations of the lower leg, right behind diabetes, which is first. Both diabetes and PVD cause loss of circulation to the lower extremities, thus increasing the risk for amputations.

According to the Center for Disease Control and Prevention, people who smoke 1½ packs of cigarettes per day or more are most likely to develop Buerger's disease. This disease can occur in people who use other forms of tobacco, like chewing tobacco. So what is Buerger's Disease? It is a disease affecting blood vessels in the arms and legs. Blood vessels swell, which can prevent blood flow causing clots to form. This can lead to pain, tissue damage, and even gangrene (the death or decay of body tissues). In some cases, amputation is required.

The most common symptoms of Buerger's disease are:

- Pale, red, or bluish hands or feet
- Cold hands or feet
- Pain in the hands and feet; may be severe

- Pain in the legs, ankles, or feet when walking—often located in the arch of the foot
- Skin changes, painful sores, or ulcers on the hands or feet

If you are a smoker, quit! Smoking leads to poor circulation and amputation. It negatively impacts healing after surgery and your ability to improve function, which can lead to further limb loss. Quitting is much less traumatic than losing a limb. That said, tobacco use is extremely addictive, and quitting is a huge challenge. Work with your physician to find a medication protocol that helps with stopping tobacco use. Seek out support from anti-smoking organizations such as the American Heart and Lung Association. Sign up for Tobacco Cessation programs in your area. Give hypnosis a try. And seek out family support. Not smoking is the most impactful activity you can do to prevent amputations.

Trauma

After Peripheral Vascular Disease, the second leading cause of limb loss is trauma. Contrary to popular belief, the leading causes of traumatic injuries are not due to war. Instead, the most common cause of traumatic amputations is motorcycle accidents. This is followed by industrial accidents, motor vehicle accidents, and falls.

Many patients are aware of their pending amputation—after multiple failed "salvage" attempts, they recognize their limb cannot be saved. Others are injured so severely that they require emergency amputations and awake in the hospital to learn of their lost limb.

Sepsis

The Sepsis Alliance defines sepsis as the body's overwhelming and life-threatening response to infection that can lead to tissue damage, organ failure, and death. In other words, it's your body's overactive and toxic response to an infection.

Your immune system usually works to fight any germs (bacteria, viruses, fungi, or parasites) to prevent infection. If an infection does occur, your immune system will try to fight it, although you may need help with medications such as antibiotics, antivirals, antifungals, and antiparasitics. However, for reasons researchers don't understand, sometimes the immune system stops fighting the "invaders" and begins to turn on itself. This is the start of sepsis.

When someone has sepsis, the blood clotting mechanism begins to work overtime. Tiny blood clots form throughout the blood system, making it difficult for blood to get to the body's organs and tissues. As the small blood clots add up, they can block the blood vessels completely.

As nutrients cannot get to the tissues in the fingers, hands, arms, toes, feet, and legs, the skin begins to die and develops gangrene. Dead tissue must be removed to stop the spread of infection, and if the damage is extensive, an amputation is necessary.

Sepsis can progress rapidly and if not treated quickly, often leads to death. As the body fights the disease, the surgeons monitor the body's response and will determine if or when an amputation is medically necessary to save the patient's life. Sepsis usually impacts all extremities and may lead to more than one limb needing to be amputated. Later on in this book, one patient will share her story of surviving sepsis.

Cancer

Amputations due to cancer are rare, with less than 2% of amputations being caused by this. The most common cancer to result in an amputated limb is osteosarcoma (bone cancer). There are less than 20,000 cases of osteosarcoma in the United States per year, and it usually occurs in teens and young adults. The survival rate is higher when the tumor is localized. When amputation is used to treat osteosarcoma cancers, the surgeon removes the portion of the limb containing the tumor including some healthy tissue above the tumor and everything below the tumor.

The goal of amputation in these cases is to remove the entire tumor and prevent any spread of the disease—again the surgery performed is to save the patient's life—providing a treatment option to recover from cancer. All patients should have detailed discussions with their doctors about treatment options available before making this weighty decision. (This book only provides information regarding cancer and how it relates to amputations, not an endorsement for any particular cancer treatment.)

Congenital Amputations

Our final segment discusses congenital amputation—a diagnosis that involves a baby being born without a limb(s) and/or being born with a deformed limb(s). It is estimated that one in 2000 babies are born each year with a missing or deformed limb. There is no known cause of congenital amputation, and there are multiple factors (genetic or environmental) that can cause a congenital amputation.

In rare instances, environmental factors can cause congenital amputation in large groups of people. Some readers may remember when many pregnant mothers were given a tranquilizer that contained the harmful drug thalidomide back in the '60s, which produced an increase in children born without limbs. Another example is the 1986 Chernobyl catastrophe in Ukraine where the radiation exposure caused many children to be born with abnormal or missing limbs. Thankfully, these are limited catastrophic events, and congenital amputations remain a very small cause of limb loss.

Understanding how a specific disease leads to limb loss is helpful in a patient's recovery. We are going to discuss the diagnoses and their reasons for amputations more specifically in upcoming chapters. Now that we understand the potential causes of amputation we are ready to discuss the different types of amputations performed.

CHAPTER 2

Types of Amputations

Now that you have a better understanding of the reasons for an amputation, it is time to discuss the different types of amputations and some of the terminology that is used to describe them. Each type creates its own set of barriers or benefits depending on the area affected.

The progression of an individual's illness is the determining factor in the level of amputation required to save his or her life. The optimal goal in every surgery is to minimize the loss of limb length. The bigger the saved portion of the limb, the easier to regain function. Remember, amputation is a lifesaving measure. The surgeon will determine the healthiest, lifesaving level of amputation that is feasible. If possible, prior to an operation, patients should discuss the probable levels limb loss with the surgeon.

This book is helpful pre-operatively as learning about the different types of amputations in advance will assist you and your physician in the discussion of the best surgery for you and in preparing for recovery. The personal stories provided will help demonstrate the difficult decisions that some have had to make. It is important to understand where your amputation needs to occur as this will also assist you through recovery. The level of your amputation has a direct correlation to how much additional energy is necessary to walk with a prosthetic limb. (Energy levels are discussed later in the book.)

Amputation levels with their medical terms and descriptions:

Partial toe	Excision of any part of one or more toes
Toe disarticulation	Disarticulation at the MTP joint
Partial foot/ray resection	Resection of 3rd–5th metatarsal and digit
Transmetatarsal	Amputation through the midsection of all metatarsals
Syme's	Ankle disarticulation with attachment of heel pad to distal of tibia
Long transtibial (Below knee)	More than 50% tibial length
Short transtibial (Below knee)	Between 20% and 50% of tibial length
Knee disarticulation	Through knee joint
Long transfemoral (Above knee)	More than 60% femoral length
Transfemoral (Above knee)	Between 35% and 60% femoral length
Short transfemoral (Above knee)	Less than 35% femoral length
Hip disarticulation	Amputation through hip joint, pelvis intact
Hemipel vectomy	Resection of lower half of the pelvis
Hemicorporectonny /Translumbar	Amputation both lower limb and pelvis below L4–L5 level

Levels of lower extremity amputations include:

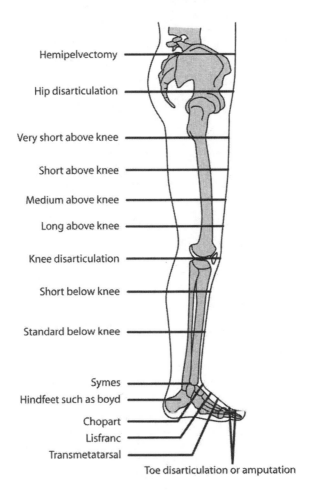

Prior to your surgery, you will undergo tests to determine how well your blood flows to your limbs. This provides the most important information to your surgeon as to which level of amputation provides the best recovery from your surgery. This is true for all vascular patients, trauma patients, and often cancer patients. Cancer patients have the added consideration of where their cancer/tumor is located.

If your surgery is planned, please consider a consultation with a physician specializing in prosthetics—usually a physiatrist also known as a Physical Medicine and Rehabilitation physician. The physiatrist understands prosthetic fitting, and this consultation will provide beneficial results towards selecting the best level of amputation and future prosthetic fittings. As always, your current state of health and the progression of your disease are the primary decision makers.

To sum up, the level of amputation required is specific to a person's medical issue, the progression of the disease, and the required recovery. Understanding the level of amputation, the why and the where, helps to prepare a patient and help them recover from your surgery.

CHAPTER 3

Personal Stories

In this chapter, several personal stories highlight the diagnoses associated with amputation. Each of these experiences is used to illustrate valuable lessons—helping you navigate your own journey, even if the related diagnosis is different than yours. Common threads of understanding can be taken from each, no matter the circumstance surrounding the loss.

As you will see, the amputees each struggled at different stages of their individual diagnosis and subsequent medical treatments. Some knew of the impending amputation while others had no knowledge (learning of their limb loss after waking up from surgery). It is a diverse group in terms of ages, cultural backgrounds, health conditions, physical conditions, and life phases. All of the amputees featured were successful with their personal goals of returning to their former lives, with some adaptations of course. And all provide inspiring information to help you and your families.

Diabetes

Larry: Bilateral Below the Knee Amputee Due to Diabetes
Larry, a diabetic amputee, lost his leg below the knee as a result of ulcers to his feet. These ulcers developed because of poor sensation due to neuropathy. He is happy to share his story and successes.

Larry was born and raised in a small town in Oklahoma. He calls himself "just a country boy who does things the country way." Larry considers himself one of the lucky ones as he was able to get out of this poor area where there was little employment for young men. One day, Larry left Oklahoma by boarding a Greyhound bus and moved to California seeking work. Within two days he had a job working in the lumber industry where he continued to work for 32 years.

In 1973, Larry met his wife through her cousin and they married in 1975. Larry and Dorothy had two children. Larry says their lives are full of lots of grandchildren and great-grandchildren. He was diagnosed with diabetes and was managing his disease with no complications for awhile. Unfortunately, the diabetes progressed over time even with good self-care. In 2004, he developed a sore on his right little toe. Larry was in a lot of pain, and he wasn't able to put his right leg on the floor. The doctors prescribed all sorts of medications, but none helped his sore toe to heal. The doctor told Larry he would need an amputation in order to heal. According to Larry, his first thought when he learned he was going to lose his leg "was no thought at all." He was in pain, and Larry wanted to walk again. His only thought about the upcoming amputation was his hope of returning to walking and being pain-free. For him there was no "decision." He wanted the surgery. Larry underwent his amputation at the below the knee level.

A short while later the same thing happened on his left foot. His second amputation was 1.5 years after the first. When Larry learned he was going to need the amputation on his left leg he used humor to accept the fact he was going to be a bilateral amputee. He recounts, "I knew I wasn't going to be growing any legs anytime soon and that was the way it was going to be." In 2006, Larry became a bilateral, below the knee amputee. Sadly, statistics show that diabetic patients that undergo an amputation are likely to need an amputation of their other leg within the next five years.

Diabetes is a progressive disease. Managed by medications, physical activity, diet, education, and by monitoring blood sugars diabetes may still lead to amputation of a limb. As Larry demonstrates later in this book, however, amputations of both his lower legs did not stop him from living his life actively and with passion.

Arteriosclerosis and Blood Clots (Thrombosis)

Carlos: Right Above the Knee Amputation Due to Arteriosclerosis and Blood Clots

Carlos from Loomis California tells us his story of losing his right leg above the knee due to arteriosclerosis and blood clots. Carlos is a non-smoker, and his story is an example of how quickly blood clots (PVD) can become a life-threatening disease. After graduating high school, Carlos enlisted in the military. Carlos spent 20 years in the military service and then chose to retire and pursue a different career. He next went to work at a hospital as a security officer for many years and then decided to change careers again. This time around he became a mechanic and went to work for Pride Industries. The mechanics contract expired, but Carlos remained at Pride Industries for the rest of his career working as a manager over several departments.

Carlos always had a love of giving back to people with disabilities. This started for him as early as high school when he volunteered and worked with special needs children. His love of working with the disabled population continued throughout his career. He also enjoyed working as a baseball umpire. Carlos will be the first to tell you he was happy and had a full life with his wife, children, and grandchildren.

One morning in July 2009, Carlos was out having breakfast with his mother. As soon as he got home, he started noticing pain in his right leg. First, Carlos tried to elevate his right leg hoping the pain would subside. Then he tried taking a hot shower to see if the heat would relax his muscles and decrease the pain, but his pain worsened. Carlos had never experienced this type of pain, and as it continued to worsen—becoming unbearable—he decided he best get to the hospital. Although his son was home, Carlos decided to drive himself. As he got into his car, Carlos realized he was unable to use his right leg, thus unable to use the pedals. He called his son on his cell phone from inside his car (his son was in the house). Carlos's son ran out to the car and drove his dad to the emergency room. In the ER, Carlos was sedated, but the pain was still the worst pain he had ever felt in his life. After two hours at the local hospital ER, Carlos was transferred by ambulance to UCD (University of California, Davis) Health Emergency Department. Carlos does not recall anything that occurred after the ambulance ride and his subsequent arrival at UCD Health.

When Carlos awoke, the pain was gone. He reached down to feel his right leg and realized part of his leg was missing; he had undergone an above knee amputation. Within 24 hours from the initial pain his right leg was completely gone. Due to a huge blood clot in his right leg, Carlos required emergency surgery. The doctors also found two smaller clots in his left leg and were able to successfully save it during the surgery. Carlos never had an opportunity to discuss his options before the surgery. The doctors informed Carlos that his right leg had a football size blood clot, and the above the knee amputation saved his life.

Carlos is an unusual case of requiring such an emergent, life-altering surgery. The majority of patients with blood clots and hardening of arteries will develop symptoms of pain and coldness and/or numbness in their affected limb followed by a visit to a vascular surgeon.

As the symptoms worsen, the patient will likely have time to discuss the need for an amputation and have undergone tests on their blood flow. Carlos's story, however, helps us understand how quickly a disease can progress, undetected, and result in a life-saving amputation.

Sepsis

Carol: Quadrilateral Amputee with Bilateral Below Knee and Bilateral Below Elbow Amputations Due to Sepsis

Carol is a born Californian with a love for the country life. Carol's love for animals led her to considered going into some type of animal science career, which is how she ended up at the University of California, Davis campus. Like many of us, Carol's career path went a different direction once in college, and she switched gears choosing to major in English. Always active, Carol decided to join a water skiing group, and this group met every weekend on the Sacramento River, which is where she met her future husband, Jim. They married three years later, started a family, and moved to Lodi where they have a small, family ranch. Carol says her life was typical, with ups and downs, but she was happy and settled. Carol was excited when she and Jim started moving into their retirement years. And then, as Carol says, "don't we get blindsided sometimes?"

On a pretty spring morning in March 2008, Carol awoke feeling perfectly fine and went on to enjoy the morning. She picked up her teenage grandchildren after school and took them for some fast food. That is the last thing she remembers. Carol, unknowingly, had an infection that was on its way toward sepsis.

Though she doesn't remember, Carol was later told that she had complained of feeling like "I might be coming down with something" and asked the grandkids' dad to come and get them just in case she was contagious. The symptoms intensified rapidly, and by the early evening, Carol was in the emergency room where they found that her vital organs were shutting down, the circulation to her extremities was restricted, and Toxic Shock (sepsis) had set in.

The culprit was a streptococcal infection. It is a pretty common organism that our bodies usually fight off. For some reason, Carol's body was overwhelmed and couldn't fight it. No one understands where Carol's strep came from. Although it attacked her internally, it was not foodborne or waterborne. What happened in this case was uncommon—beyond the talent and resources of the local hospital. A doctor even suggested to her family that they say their goodbyes, that there was nothing more to be done. Although he had never met Carol or her family, the physician told her family that Carol had had a good life, and if she did survive, she would suffer the loss of both her hands and both her feet. The physician went on to tell them that no one would want to live with those disabilities.

Carol's family is very tough by nature. Yes, Carol's life had been good, but they knew she would choose life with disabilities over death. While Carol was in a coma and sleeping through the critical days, they fought (and it was a fight) to get her released from an inadequate hospital and admitted to UC Davis Health where so many talented and dedicated doctors and medical professionals believed that they could give Carol a good life. And they worked very hard to make that happen. As Carol started to recover, she was able to see the damage to her limbs. She had to wait weeks until she was healthy enough to have the surgeries.

Carol knew she was scheduled to have her arms and legs amputated, but she was determined to live. She admits that she didn't really know what her life was going to be like, but she knew she wanted one so she had both arms amputated below the elbow, and both legs amputated below the knee.

Sepsis is a fast moving, often deadly, infectious disease. Our bodies fight hard to survive giving up our limbs so we can live. The amputations due to sepsis are not only lifesaving, but also assist with healing and can lead to better prosthetic devices to improve the patient's quality of life. Carol certainly has determination, survival instincts, deep faith, and a loving, supportive family. Her story will certainly inspire all of us to achieve our goals.

Cancer

Ray: Right Hip Disarticulation Due to Cancer
Ray is excited to share his cancer survivor story and he does have a long, complicated story to tell! Ray is a native Californian, born in Long Beach in 1953. Ray's parents died at an early age due to congestive heart failure, and he committed to himself to lead a healthy lifestyle. Ray was always a go-getter. Starting in 4th grade, Ray raised animals at home. At age 11, he started his career as an entrepreneur. And at age 14, Ray went to work at a Mobil gas station—becoming manager within three months.

Ray's personal and work life moved forward with college, marriage, divorce and successful, entrepreneurial career moves. In the summer of 2004, Ray decided to visit his sister in Southern California for a holiday. While visiting, the family decided to go to an amusement park for the day. While on a bumpy rollercoaster ride, Ray felt a "pop" in his back. He thought it was just a pulled muscle and ignored the pain. Ray kept waiting for the "muscle spasm" to get better, but after several months it was actually getting worse. His left leg started dragging, and the pain was increasing. It was time to go to the doctor.

X-rays were ordered. Ray went to have the x-rays taken, and while actually on the x-ray machine, a technician frantically came into the room. He told Ray not to move as Ray was transferred onto a stretcher and taken to a top level 1 trauma center hospital in Northern California for an urgent MRI. During the next 72 hours, Ray was poked, prodded, and tested multiple times, but no one told him what was happening. He finally couldn't take it and had a panic attack—what was going on?

Finally, Ray was told the devastating news, "Ray you have Stage 4 cancer and it is all over your body. It has deteriorated all your bones in the body, which are now like eggshells. If you fall, you could break all the bones in your body." His hip had fractured on the park ride. Ray was told there was nothing to be done and he was only given a few weeks to live.

The next step was to be seen by an orthopedic oncologist, and this physician agreed to take his case. His words to Ray—

"You're not going to die. You will go through hell and back, but you are not going to die." Ray was admitted to the hospital in Berkeley, California for a long, hospital stay. The first step to initiate treatment was to determine the exact type of cancer Ray had. The test required tissue being removed by a needle from Ray's left hip, but during the test Ray's hip collapsed into pieces. The good news: the cancer was easy to treat. The bad news: he needed to have his hip repaired. After the hip replacement surgery, Ray would need extensive radiation and chemotherapy. He stayed at the hospital in Berkeley for a full year. The treatment was not over after that however, and trying to survive cancer was not making Ray's life any easier.

After a year in the hospital, Ray returned to Sacramento, California to finish up his cancer treatments. It was AWFUL!! Each time he went for a chemotherapy session, he would develop a neutropenic fever. He became so ill that his hospitalization included isolation and a course of intravenous antibiotics. Then he would return back home for injections into his abdomen every eight hours. During this arduous journey, Ray was determined to walk. He began with a walker on his new left hip replacement and immediately had tremendous, hip pain—way more than the innocuous pain that started this journey back on the rollercoaster. So Ray went back to the hospital for hip surgery. During surgery, it became apparent that his hip joint was infected, and that Ray was going to have to have a second hip replacement. Unfortunately, the outcome was not good, and his second hip replacement became infected also. An additional surgery was required with antibiotics surgically placed into his left hip joint in the form of beads.

Ray was ready to go home after surgery number three and started driving when his cell phone rang. It was his surgeon, "Stop. Turn around and carefully drive back to the hospital. Your hip is in pieces, and you need a fourth surgery." Ray was discouraged—he turned around and returned to the hospital, and had the fourth hip replacement. This time, Ray improved, he began feeling "human" again gaining strength and progressing in his walking. Ray was improving so well that he began to transition to a cane.

And then, suddenly, he felt the all too familiar pain again in his left hip. Ray termed this pain "The Big One." Sepsis had set in. The doctors gathered together and informed Ray at best he had a month to live. They recommended he go to a convalescent home and hospice care for the remainder of his life.

Seven months later...

Ray was still in the convalescence home. He was supposed to be dead, but instead he was walking the halls with a walker and machines attached to his hip (wound vacs). Ray wasn't ready to die, and he certainly wasn't going to die in a convalescent home.

Ray was told he could not be discharged because he was too sick so Ray planned his escape. He started watching the nurses and their shift changes—checking for when the doorways were not staffed. Three weeks later Ray went into action. A close friend pulled up to the home at 2:30 a.m. and Ray walked out of the doors and went home. Immediately, his health started to improve. Ray contacted a home health, nursing agency and soon nurses were coming to his home. His infection control physician came to Ray's home to check on him and was pleased with his progress. Ray was right; dying was not on his schedule.

Ray's health took the long road to recovery. First, his body negatively reacted to the medication and his kidneys began to fail. Return to the hospital was imminent. Ray decided he needed something to look forward to so just before he went into the hospital he decided to buy himself a new car. No matter what the doctors told him, and no matter what the treatment was going to be, once out of the hospital, Ray was going to have something to look forward to doing, which was driving his new car. He again looked at his calendar and, "Nope, dying was not on my schedule." He just knew he was going to beat cancer and sepsis.

Once admitted to the hospital, the news was again grim. His only chance to live was to amputate his left leg. This was not as easy of a decision for Ray as many people might think. He had gone through four hip replacements, years of cancer treatment, and seven horrible months in a nursing facility. All his energy had been focused on walking and saving his left limb. He didn't want to "give up" the fight to save his leg, and he was feeling disappointed and depressed.

Two months went by and again the physicians told Ray, "We must amputate your left leg for you to live." The doctors gave him less than a week to live, and he needed the surgery immediately. Ray thought, "I'm not ready to die, I want to live, I am expecting another grandchild, and I need to live for my family." The doctors told Ray he would be confined to a wheelchair never able to walk again. Ray was sure he wanted to live, but was concerned about losing his leg and his ability to walk. What kind of life would it be to not be able to walk?

In the end, Ray chose to live. He told the physician on a Tuesday, had the amputation on a Thursday, and on Friday he woke up feeling amazing—No pain! Ray wasn't taking any pain medication—he felt GREAT! He asked the doctor how much of his leg they took. His reply was, "All of it and two ribs." Ray's left lower limb amputation was at the second highest level—a hip disarticulation.

After such a long and arduous journey starting with a horrific cancer diagnosis, followed by sepsis, and a hip disarticulation amputation, all of us would understand if Ray had had enough. As you have figured out by the point, however, it was not in Ray's nature to give up. Instead, he found his way back to living his life.

Trauma

Jon: Right Knee Disarticulation Due to Trauma
Jon was born in 1974 at Sutter Memorial Hospital and grew up in Rancho Cordova, California with his brother, his dad, and his stepmom. Jon went to Cordova High School and graduated in 1992. He was always involved in sports, playing soccer at age four, and starting wrestling in the 8th grade. Jon wrestled all through high school and then at Sacramento City College. Jon enrolled in college, but only so he could continue wrestling. Throughout his teen years, Jon had a lot of different jobs and considers beginning his real career at age 21 with a local utility company. Jon met his wife in 2001—a waitress at a Filipino restaurant—Jon loves the story of how he met his wife. He walked into the restaurant to have lunch, and as soon as he saw the waitress, he knew she was the one! After

much convincing, the waitress agreed to go out on a date, and they have now been married 16 years and have three children.

The year 2001 was a big one for Jon as he had met his wife and was working full time for the utility company as a lineman. His life was very busy with a lot of hours climbing poles, crawling under houses, going up into attics, dropping lines into residential homes. That year, he also bought a house, a Harley, and he resumed playing soccer in adult leagues. Jon was happy, proud of his accomplishments, and looking forward to his future.

Jon had been with the same company for nine years, and the company was going through many changes. He also felt ready for a change as he had an opportunity to move to another utility company working a similar job. After passing the written test, Jon was invited to a two-day climbing school where the students are evaluated. Only eighteen trainees from Jon's group were invited to the advanced, two-week training, and Jon was one of them. The passing rate is only 25%, so out of the eighteen invitees only 4-5 trainees would likely be hired.

Jon was confident he would be able to pass the training as his current job was so similar to the new job he was training for. By the final day, only four of the original eighteen were still in the training program. To be hired, they needed to pass a final, timed trial. Jon volunteered to go first as he didn't want to deal with the stress of waiting. To pass, he needed to complete the test within 45 minutes, but to get the job he needed to beat that time. The task had to be done correctly as well as be under the required time. Once completing the task of building the test equipment, the test is over, but then you have to disassemble the equipment and lower it back to the ground.

Jon had been working lineman jobs for nine years, and historically, his legs tended to consistently go numb if he was up on the line for an extended period. Jon was used to his legs going numb. He was not surprised that his left leg was numb just as he completed sending the equipment to the ground. He had no idea what his time was, and he wanted to hustle to get down the pole to finish and pass the test. Unbeknownst to Jon, once the equipment hit the ground, the test ended. He believed he still needed to touch the ground for the test to end. After two weeks of intense training, and using all his annual vacation time, Jon was determined to pass the test. He came straight down the pole, landing flat-footed on bark chips as he fell to the ground. He was conscious the entire time and knew something horrible had happened to his leg. It felt like a car was sitting on top of his leg, and the pressure just kept building and building.

He asked three times what his timed test result was—it was so important to Jon to know if he passed the test and if all his hard work was coming to fruition. He wanted to be one of the few that could succeed and get the job. Finally, the examiner told him he was under 36 minutes—he felt immediate relief. He was going to be able to get a new job! But the leg pain was still there and became his focus. Jon had no idea how serious his leg injury was even with the severe pain he was feeling.

Someone called an ambulance, but the training site was out in the county, down back roads. By the time the ambulance arrived, 30 minutes had passed since the accident. Then it was an additional 45-60 minutes to get to the hospital. Jon was given IV pain medication, but there was no relief, and he was feeling worse with each passing moment. When he finally arrived at the UCD Health emergency room, he was aware that something really bad had happened to his leg. The doctor adjusted his IV in the ER, and Jon was "out like a light."

In the hospital, Jon learned the fall had snapped the femoral artery in his right leg, but he had no injuries that broke through his skin.

This meant his artery was bleeding into his leg, which was swelling; he needed emergent surgery. Jon had a total of five surgeries in three days with the first four surgeries attempting to repair the femoral artery. Those three days were the worst three days of his entire life.

The pain in his right leg was constant and severe; he was unable to sleep or eat due to all the scheduled surgeries. After days of unsuccessful surgeries, Jon's lower leg was slowly dying. The swelling in his lower leg, called compartment syndrome, resulted in his knee being "filleted" open, to manage the swelling. Jon could see his leg was not recovering. The physician finally told Jon he was going to need an amputation to which Jon wasn't surprised. His immediate concern became, "How am I going to tell my family?" unaware that the doctor had already taken care of that.

Jon's fifth and final surgery was finally completed—a knee disarticulation, also known as a through knee amputation. Jon says he awoke for the first time from the surgery with a magical relief from the pain. The immediate pain relief was huge for Jon. He knew the surgery was the right medical decision and he felt positive about his recovery.

Jake: Bilateral Below the Knee Amputations Due to Trauma
Born in San Jose and raised in Fair Oaks California, Jake grew up "just a normal kid." He was very athletic and played sports throughout school. After high school, Jake went to UC Berkeley as a walk-on for the football team, which is very difficult to achieve. Jake was even able to earn a football scholarship! After several years of college, Jake was still unsure of what he wanted out of life so he made a huge decision to drop out of college and travel for a year—going as far as China. When returning home, Jake finished college, earning his degree. As his career developed, Jake took a position working 6-month rotations between the North Pole and Antarctica—setting up research field camps and preparing the area for the scientists who would come in later to perform their research

projects. Jake was working a summer in Greenland where he enjoyed his work and was happy. His specific job contributed to providing the world a better understanding of atmospheric changes and climate change. He couldn't imagine being any happier.

On one particular day, knowing a storm was coming, he and his coworker went out to secure the sites, as Jake says to "batten down the hatches." They were about three miles out of camp when the storm came on suddenly and hard. Jake and his coworker became separated. The storm quickly became more violent and turned into a complete whiteout.

Jake could not even see his hand in front of his face so he had to "hunker down" in the storm, alone, for three days and three nights. Just like a scene in a movie, Jake had to stay awake and fight off hypothermia. He battled it successfully, being able to finally make his way back to camp. All along the way, Jake kept thinking to himself that he was probably going to lose a few fingers and toes, which goes along with the job. He always knew this risk was a possibility in his line of work, but his 17 years of experience provided him all the skills necessary to survive. He followed a search plane and walked himself halfway back to camp; he was able to flag down a snowcat and was picked up by his co-workers. Jake was immediately helicoptered to the closest hospital in Greenland in the capital city Nuuk. He was hospitalized there for one week and then flown back to the United States to UCD Health in Sacramento, California. Jake remembers waking up after his first night at UC Davis Health and his right hand was gone. Next, began the slow process of trying to save his feet.

When all was said and done, Jake underwent seven different amputations, all were attempts to try and save his legs. Jake was advised to consider bilateral below knee amputations. This included in-depth discussions, which permitted Jake and his wife time to process and understand the benefits of this type of surgery. After a couple of days of considering his options, Jake made the easy decision to go ahead with the surgery—a decision he has never regretted. Jake understood clearly that the amputations would provide him the functionality he desired.

Forty-five percent of all amputations are due to trauma. This is an incredibly life changing event, to be so severely injured that you require a lifesaving procedure as dramatic as an amputation. Jake's amputations, like the others in this book, however, allowed him to live a more functional life rather than continuing to struggle with his injured limbs.

Congenital Abnormality

Megan: Below the Knee Amputation Due to Congenital Abnormality
Megan was not born without limbs, but due to a congenital defect, she required an amputation during her teenage years. Megan was born with a small benign tumor on her spine—a small belly button on her lower back as her mother describes. At three months of age, Megan underwent surgery to remove the tumor, and the surgery was a success. She grew up as a "normal" Californian in the Bay area. Throughout her growing years, Megan did notice she tolerated walking on rocks/gravel without any pain or difficulty, which was due to decreased sensation in her feet. As a kid, you are not aware of deficits, especially decreased sensation in your feet as you have no experiences to compare it to. Megan had no real issues with her feet during her childhood, playing soccer and sports and other normal kid stuff.

Then one day while running in her backyard, Megan fell and broke her foot—she wore a cast and then a walking boot, but her foot would not heal. This was the first, real indication that there was something not normal about her feet. She went to the doctor, and that is where she learned that she had poor circulation in her feet, especially in the left foot after the fracture occurred. She was starting to lose function in her foot so the next step was surgery, but her foot would still not heal. Further investigation by the doctors led them to her back. The scar tissue from her childhood surgery had grown around her spine and was now pinching her spine causing nerve damage in the form of lack of sensation and lack of circulation to her leg. She was diagnosed with "tethered spine," which is not an uncommon diagnosis, but unfamiliar to Megan and her family.

Megan continued with her life on a bum foot. It didn't seem to interfere much, and she started to resume her activities as best she could. Over time, her left leg progressively worsened. At first she noticed her leg starting to look different. Then her foot started to lose mobility and strength, and she wasn't able to move her foot up and down. She began to feel like it was a club foot and she noticed she really couldn't use her foot like normal people. She started tripping frequently. At 17 she went to a surgeon who unaware of how little Megan and her family understood of her diagnosis bluntly informed her she was going to need an amputation. She was stunned by the news. The physician referred her to an orthopedic surgeon for a consultation, but she decided to try some other options first using different braces to help her walk. The poor sensation in her foot, however, led to sores and ulcers from the braces. Megan's issues were very similar to what diabetics face.

Megan remembers the impact of her left foot's poor functionality. She was a teenager and wanted to be active, but she was becoming more and more sedentary. She was no longer playing sports or even able to participate in her physical education class. After graduating high school and starting her first year in college, Megan had difficulty just walking to classes. She was continuing to trip frequently and was embarrassed in front of her classmates. It was time for Megan to evaluate her physical limitations and come to a decision.

Painfully, Megan and her family sat down and discussed the pros and cons of having an amputation. Going on the internet to do "research," Megan first saw a story about Heather Mills and her Dancing with the Stars Fame. Megan was excited to see how beautiful Heather's prosthetic legs were, especially the skin. She felt relieved that her leg would look more normal than she expected, even being able to wear regular shoes including strappy sandals and high heels.

While her primary information source was the internet, Megan did meet with an orthopedic surgeon to learn more about the procedure and outcomes. She also met with a prosthetist who gave her a CD with information about becoming an amputee, and he put her in email contact with another female amputee. Megan contacted the young woman, and they shared emails, but did not meet until several years later. She did meet briefly with a counselor to discuss her feelings though she admits the session was not as needed as she thought—after 5-6 years of dealing with a bum foot, she was ready for a potentially life-improving procedure. The amputation offered her an opportunity to gain more functionality with her life instead of dealing with bulky braces and limited mobility. Megan underwent a below the knee amputation.

While Megan's story isn't exactly the same as being born with absent or deformed limbs, it does represent a young child born with a disability who then chooses amputation during her teenage years to improve her quality of life. A child born with a congenital amputation will learn through activity and development what works best for them in their ever changing future. Parents have the chance to work with the medical team to provide the best opportunities for their child's physical and emotional development.

PART II

Recovery Phases after an Amputation

CHAPTER 4

Reacting to the News

In the area of emotional responses to amputation, there is no hard and fast research to cite. However, through my years of experience working in this field, I have identified some patterns that are worth sharing. There are no "correct" reactions, and all feelings are normal. All amputees go through ups and downs with their emotions. There is no timeline for emotional recovery.

Many patients who experience limb loss go through the same stages of grief as those experiencing death and dying. In 1969 Dr. Elizabeth Kubler-Ross introduced the stages of dying in her book, *On Death and Dying*. The five stages she identified are: denial, anger, bargaining, depression, and acceptance. All five stages are a natural part of the grieving process and are a framework that we use to help identify what we may be feeling as we experience traumatic loss.

These stages are not linear, and amputees will go in and out of stages or even skip some stages altogether. Psychologists reaffirm that there is no "correct emotional response" to an amputation. All feelings are healthy, normal, and should not be judged by anyone. How patients and caregivers respond to their amputation depends upon their unique make-up (personality, values, & attitudes), previous life experiences, current support systems, and the meaning they attach to their amputation.

Amputees that suffered significant pain before their surgery and are aware of the pending surgery often have feelings of relief. They have suffered to the point where their lives were negatively impacted by pain and limited mobility. Almost all of my patients that had multiple surgeries in an attempt to save their leg report to me that they wish they could have just started with the amputation surgery and moved on with their lives. Those with vascular disease report pain relief and are excited they are going to be able to walk again with a prosthetic limb. I am often asked by patients if this is normal—this feeling of relief, of progress and optimism. Yes, it is normal, more often than not. Feeling better is normal and no amputee should feel crazy for thinking that.

Amputees that suffer a traumatic amputation and wake up to suddenly learn of their limb loss are the patients who more typically experience stages of grief. Interestingly though, my observations with these patients as a whole is how goal-oriented they are towards returning to walking. This population typically does not have compromising medical conditions and are generally motivated to "get to work." They do excellent with a plan of action and even better when they understand the process ahead. Their focus is all about the rehabilitation—while their emotional processing is usually set aside to work on their physical goals. Once they achieve their physical goals and return home is when the emotional challenges and stages of grief seem to begin.

If you are about to go through an amputation or if you have just experienced one, remember you are not alone! You are not the only person to lose a limb, and you will get through this stage of your life. Ask for help. Many of my clients will seek out counseling—which is wonderful. I recommend you find a psychologist or social worker with a background in rehabilitation. Search out amputee support groups in your area. Try multiple support groups to find a group that fits your needs. Look into your area's disabled sports groups. Find an amputee peer that you can talk to. Often your medical team can find a peer for you to meet. Amputee Coalition is a group which provides amputees information regarding groups and peer support and can be found online. Books are also a great resource. I recommend a self-guided book called *Bouncing Back: Skills for Adaptation to Injury, Aging, Illness, and Pain* by Richard Wanlass, Ph.D. (http://www.amazon.com/dp/0190610557/) A list of support resources is also listed at the end of this segment.

During your rehabilitation, work with your medical team to set realistic goals for yourself. Everyone wants to walk, but understanding the physical challenges and your medical limitations will help you recognize the steps and the processes required to get you back to walking. Start with small and simple, short-term goals like first learning how to successfully don your prosthesis. Too often the long-term goals that are set such as "walking" are too far off or too general to be motivating. These goals need to be broken down into smaller, short-term targets like being able to walk in your home with a walker. The ultimate, long-term goal may be to walk with a cane inside your home or even outside your home, but the first, short-term objective gives you something to aim at immediately, which motivates you to keep moving toward your ultimate goal.

Just as a baby learns to crawl before standing and then moves to walking, amputees must progress through similar stages to get to their long-term goals. Do not compare yourself to others—no two people are alike! Appreciate how your body still works for you. Recognize what you have rather than what you have lost. Consider the strength it took to get as far as you have along the way and give yourself well-deserved credit for getting there.

All of the amputees in this book had different reactions and responses when learning about their amputations. Some grieved and some were relieved. Others were depressed. And some were actually invigorated to move to the next step of rehab. Let's take a look at how the amputees from Section One emotionally handled their different situations. You may be able to identify with some or all of them during the different stages of their grief and relief.

Carol: Quadrilateral Amputee with Bilateral Below Knee and Bilateral Below Elbow Amputations Due to Sepsis

Carol the sepsis survivor understood the general assumption that losing all four limbs creates a total loss of independence and a high demand from loved ones. Carol knew she was going to have the surgery and lose all her limbs, but as Carol reported in her story, she had a very good life. Carol always had, and still has, a firm faith in a loving God, who would get her through this. And she still feels today all the blessings that come in the form of a loving and supportive husband and family and terrific friends. As Carol transitioned, she was uncertain of her future but was still optimistic and determined to live.

One thing that is standard in hospitals is to have a psychologist visit those who have suffered a calamity. A very nice psychologist came to see Carol and puzzled over why Carol had not ever cried. The psychologist had concerns about Carol being in the stage of denial, but Carol knew that she had cheated death and that every day she was moving forward in strength and mobility. Carol was also kept busy with rehabilitation and received lots of attention in the hospital. She was getting huge support from her family and friends. Even people she barely knew reached out to her.

As Carol started showing signs of recovery, her husband reminded her in strong terms that "Everyone has been going the extra mile for you. Now you have to do your part." Carol would eventually deal with four prostheses, but her recovery started with learning how to turn over in bed. There was a lot of work to be done. Carol's attitude was that she needed to put her best effort possible into her recovery not only for herself, but also for all of those who had gone the extra mile in helping her.

After four months in the hospital, Carol was released to go home. She left the hospital in a wheelchair, and that is when reality set in. As Carol began to resume life, it definitely hit hard that her life would never be the same. Moments of grief seemed to bubble out at times as she mourned her loss. Carol's husband understood those times and they let the moments naturally happen. After a while, the moments were gone. Overall, Carol was always convinced she had the faith, family, and perseverance to get on with her life.

Ray: Right Hip Disarticulation Due to Cancer

Ray was ready to get on with his life. After his hip disarticulation, he finally felt GREAT. And proving the doctors wrong was now a habit. Ray didn't die after being given three death sentences. Now he was told he would never walk again—not this Ray. Determined to prove the doctors wrong once again, Ray "walked" out of the hospital with a walker and "hopping" on his right leg.

Soon Ray began noticing pain at the amputation site. His doctors sent him to a psychiatrist, then to an acupuncturist, and then for a trial of TENS (electrical stimulation used for pain control). His doctors told Ray that he was completely out of ideas on how to treat him, and he didn't know how to help Ray, but that a referral to PM&R (Physical Medicine and Rehabilitation) for evaluation would be helpful. Ray had no idea what PM&R was, and he had no idea what another doctor was going to offer him for his pain. Ray assumed the appointment was for his pain—but was Ray ever wrong about this appointment. His physician, Dr. Shin, asked him if he knew why he was there. Ray told him he thought it was for pain management. "No," said Dr. Shin, "We are going to fit you with a prosthesis. And you are going to walk again!" Ray was in disbelief.

What—walk again? He was overwhelmed. The GREATest words he had ever heard were, "You're going to walk again."

Jon: Right Knee Disarticulation Due to Trauma

Jon's initial trauma was severe. After multiple surgeries on his leg, the pain relief achieved post-amputation gave him the much needed confidence in his decision to amputate. Prior to the decision, however, Jon felt overwhelmed by the amount of information coming at him, and as no one plans on spending their life as an amputee, he struggled with trying to understand the information and implications for his future. Jon noted how many people were coming in to speak with him during his hospitalization. It was difficult to know his options and to understand what the physician was discussing, however he was at least able to understand that a below the knee amputation (BKA) was not an option.

One of the physicians was excited about the possibility of performing a knee disarticulation surgery also known as a through knee operation. In this procedure, the two bones that make up your lower leg, the tibia and femur, are separated at the joint. The end of the femur bone remains intact, which can later assist in support of a prosthetic. Understanding the pluses and minuses of this procedure versus a traditional above the knee amputation (AKA) was difficult to discern. Jon trusted his physicians. He was glad he was taken to a progressive hospital with a multidisciplinary team to assist him with all the decisions. The team consisted of his surgeon, PM&R physician, and physical therapist. Jon's hospitalization lasted three weeks. During this time, his family and friends readied the house for him—building ramps inside and outside his home and making his house wheelchair accessible.

Jon was discharged home in a wheelchair with a knee disarticulation, and he was very optimistic he would continue his recovery and be able to walk again. Looking back, Jon says he would not change any part of the decision to have the knee disarticulation vs. the traditional above the knee amputation.

Megan: Below the Knee Amputation Due to Congenital Abnormality

Megan, our teenage amputee, struggled after her surgery. Megan moved into her parents' home and took a semester off from college. The first two months Megan felt shut down—she stayed home, not going out. She didn't want to hang out with her friends or go out in public. She was very self-conscious and wanted to hide the fact that she was an amputee. She didn't want anyone to see her leg until she was walking. Her family was very supportive. Megan admits she could not accept her amputation the first few months. She had all the concerns and doubts all teenagers have, which was heightened by her amputation. Would her friends accept her? Would she be able to have a boyfriend and get married in the future?

Megan's self-consciousness and self-doubt started to lessen as she began walking with her prosthesis. She was able to hide her prosthesis under her pants, and she walked normally so people didn't notice she was an amputee. As she became more active, she tried going to the gym. Megan's confidence grew when at the gym she discovered she could exercise on the treadmill and elliptical, and no one noticed her lower leg!

The struggle to tell her friends she was an amputee continued though. As she slowly shared her amputation with girlfriends, they easily accepted her. Finally, she began telling the boys she dated about her prosthesis. Again, no issues ever came up. Megan states, reflecting back, her lack of confidence and insecurities were more age-related than actually being related to her amputation. The normal girl things in high school—clothing, shoes, appearance, and fitting in become less important as you mature and grow up. This happened as Megan matured and realized that her amputation was the right decision for improving her functional life having little impact on her social relationships.

Carlos: Right Above the Knee Amputation Due to Arteriosclerosis and Blood Clots

Carlos had a blood clot that required emergency surgery to save his life. He remembers waking after his surgery, feeling around with his hands and figuring out that he didn't have a lower leg. Heavily medicated, he was trying to sort out what had happened to him in the last 24 hours. A lot of thoughts raced through his minds until the physician came in and told him what happened to him. The physician told him the surgery saved his life. At that moment, Carlos felt grateful to be alive. His family felt the same way. Everyone was ready to take steps forward to return to their lives together even if it meant living life a little differently.

Carlos shared that he does have tearful moments. He cries when he realizes new limitations, but then he resets himself and converts his loss into a mission of learning a different way of doing things. Carlos has never been sad about the loss of his leg as he is just so happy to be alive. But change can be overwhelming, and he understands he needs to process his feelings in the moment before moving forward again.

Jake: Bilateral Below the Knee Amputations Due to Trauma

Jake suddenly awoke at the hospital without his right arm below the elbow. Before his next surgery though, Jake had time to process and understand that his future also included losing both legs below the knee. Jake is grateful he had an excellent team of physicians to help him understand his choices regarding additional amputations. The decision to go ahead with the bilateral below the knee amputations was a team decision including Jake, his wife, and his physicians. At the time, Jake's parents were distraught and struggled with the thought of their son losing his limbs, but they left the room and allowed Jake and his wife to make the decision that was best for them. He had been in the hospital for two months, already losing his right hand and almost his left. Jake had been through so much and was being given an opportunity to find a way to regain his functional life. Jake firmly believes that this type of decision is very individualistic and each person needs to make the decision that is best for them.

During his rehabilitation is when Jake noticed his emotions were a roller coaster of good and bad days. Questions of what he was going to be able to do started to fill his mind. His thoughts ran the gamut from suicide to wanting to be the first triple amputee to climb Mount Everest. His emotions were fully charged and at the forefront. Jake had his "game face" on when around others, but then would go home and break down. He didn't understand depression, as he had never experienced such significant life changes before, or ever knowingly been around those who suffered from depression. Jake was concerned with overburdening his wife who was also going through adjustment changes. Though Jake never considered counseling before, he felt that an outside observer—someone objective that he could talk to—would be helpful. Jake began counseling to help him manage his up and downs. Counseling had huge positive benefits for him.

Jake was suffering from Post Traumatic Stress Disorder (PTSD), which is very common with our military veterans who witnessed trauma during their tour of service. Jake described that his dreams were of his body having all his limbs, and he would awake and realize he had lost his limbs all over again. As the emotional healing began, Jake noticed his dreams had changed to include his current body. For Jake, this was a turning point. Jake believes his grieving process lasted 18-24 months. Again, Jake acknowledges that during this time, counseling was immensely helpful. Accepting himself just as he was finally moved him all the way out of the grieving process. Jake realized he could do everything he did before; he just has to do it differently. Jake emotionally and intellectually concluded that he was no longer going to blame his life changes on his amputations, and that he would be the person he saw himself being.

The emotional reactions experienced when learning you need an amputation through post-surgery and post-rehabilitation are very personal and individualized. As stated before, the stages of grief are not linear; they ebb and flow through time and experience. It is my hope that all amputees be kind to themselves, allowing appropriate time to process and emotionally recover.

To the amputees out there who feel alone, you are not! This book and other resources are available to help you see that there are many others who have experienced what you are facing and that there is hope. Give yourself credit for your small victories and be patient with the long-term goals. You are alive, and soon you will be back to living.

CHAPTER 5

Family Reactions

Your amputation does not impact you alone. Your family is also affected by your amputation. Family members will undergo their own process as they walk through some of the stages of grief and adjust to the changes that limb loss creates for them, not just for the amputee, but for the entire family's lives.

The impact of illness on the family/caregiver is often underplayed as caregivers are focused on their loved one's recovery. But the changes in their lives are real too. For example, if the patient was working prior to their amputation: Will they be able to return to work? How will the bills be paid? How will their future income be impacted? And if the caregiver is working, how will their work be affected. Will there be a need to miss a lot of work while caring for their loved one? Financial insecurity is a real stressor and should be addressed to help decrease the worry for everyone.

Caregivers will also be adjusting to any physical modifications made to the home that need completed before the patient can return such as adding a ramp for entrance into the home and potential bathroom modifications (which will be described in the next section). The caregiver will need to obtain medical equipment such as a wheelchair to help with independence when the patient first gets home. In addition, other home responsibilities may shift onto the caregiver, the most noted being driving the amputee to all of his or her medical appointments until he or she is able to return to driving.

Social issues may be a concern for caregivers and patients alike. As in our patient stories above, new amputees may be reluctant to socialize until they are further along in their rehabilitation. Family members may feel a loss of socialization as they too focus on supporting the patient during their rehabilitation. For some caregivers, their decrease in social times with friends may be difficult, and the caregiver may feel a loss of their support system.

Communication is key for caregiver and patient. The amputee is working on improving their functional lives and trying to return to a new normal. Family members will also need to accept the changing circumstances and will need information to help everyone stay focused on the short-term goals and eventually the long-term goals.

Support must be a give and take. Families want to help and assist in your adjustments, but they often have no direction on how to help you. You, the patient, need to get comfortable with stating what you need in the moment. As you recover, your needs will change especially as you regain your independence. Please be willing to talk with your caregiver about the changing roles as your rehab progresses.

Caregivers also need to focus on communication skills. Where in the stages of emotional grief are they? What are their needs and how can you, the patient, support the caregiver? This sharing, open communication is how your family relationships deepen and grow. Both patient's and family's emotional recoveries move in and out of phases and more often than not they don't keep the same pace. Take a moment to reflect on how each of you is feeling and put yourself in each other's place.

Each individual, whether caregiver or patient, brings a unique set of life experiences, values, and attitudes that they have utilized throughout their lives to deal with stress. No situation is the same so no reaction can be planned for. Being educated and informed regarding the medical condition, the surgery, and the physical and emotional requirements for healing will decrease the stress of the "unknown." The better informed everyone is, the better planning and better outcomes for all.

And just as the patient needs to remember to care for themselves, the caregiver needs to remember the same. Eat healthy, get good sleep, take time to exercise and socialize with friends. Caring for yourself, emotionally and physically, will actually improve your ability to care for your family member. The patient does not want to be a burden so support them by showing you will still be the same person, doing your same activities.

Again, none of you are alone. The same resources for amputees are also available for family members. Reach out to amputee support groups, seek out counseling, and find time for yourself. There is help available to assist with your emotional well-being during the recovery phase and after if needed. Be kind to yourselves and each other.

Resources:

Disabled Sports USA: http://www.disabledsportsusa.org/

Amputee Coalition: https://www.amputee-coalition.org/

Gold River Amputee Support Group: http://www.goldcountryamputees.com/

UCD Health Amputee Support Group:
https://www.ucdmc.ucdavis.edu/medicalcenter/patients/support_groups.html

"Bouncing Back: Skills For Adaptation To Injury, Aging, Illness, and Pain" by Richard Wanlass, Ph.D:
https://www.amazon.com/dp/0190610557

PART III

Post-Operative Phase

CHAPTER 6

The Team

Generally speaking, the period from post-hospital through the prosthetic fitting is very similar for all amputees. The timing of each step will vary dependent upon the health and healing of the patient after the amputation. The post-operative phase is also considered the rehabilitation phase. Rehabilitation begins immediately after the surgery in the hospital and is a very active phase for the patient and their family.

The rehabilitation process includes a multi-disciplinary team of health professionals to help you achieve your highest level of independence. Your team consists of the surgeon, physical therapists, occupational therapists, nurses, social workers, prosthetists, and your physiatrist (a physician specializing in rehabilitation). In detail, the roles of your team are as follows:

Surgeon

Depending on your diagnosis, you may have an orthopedic, trauma, or vascular physician. He or she performs the surgery and follows your healing process until you are ready to be fitted for a prosthetic limb.

Physical Therapist (PT)

The PT works with you to promote your ability to move, reduce pain, and start to restore your function with exercises. After you receive your prosthetic limb, your physical therapist will work with you on learning how to walk with your prosthesis.

Occupational Therapist (OT)

The OT helps you regain skills for activities of daily living, (such as bathing and dressing), provides recommendations for adaptive equipment including training in its use, and guidance and education for family members and caregivers.

Social Worker (SW)

Social workers review new admissions for issues that need addressing and assist with discharge planning. They may help patients locate various resources within their communities.

Physical Medicine and Rehabilitation Physician (Physiatrist)

The physiatrist's role is to enhance and restore functional ability and quality of life to those with physical impairments or disabilities. Physiatrists specialize in prosthetic rehabilitation and will be the doctor prescribing your prosthetic limb and following your prosthetic care.

Prosthetist

The prosthetist is the person who will make your artificial (prosthetic) limb and follow you for all your prosthetic needs.

CHAPTER 7

Hospital to Home

Inpatient

The goals of inpatient rehabilitation are to improve a patient's mobility, prevent contractures, dial in pain management, control edema, and promote healing. Contractures are the chronic losses of joint motion due to structural changes in non-bony tissue. These non-bony tissues include muscles, ligaments, and tendons.

The amputated limb will be in a post-operative dressing and for below knee amputees possibly in an open splint to keep the knee straight. The lower limb should be elevated to assist with decreasing the swelling from the surgery. Your physician and nurse will assist you with your medications for pain management. Physical Therapy and Occupational Therapy will assist in training you with transfers from your bed to a chair and bathing transfers for when you return home. Your physician will determine if you are safe to ambulate with a walker or crutches, but do not be concerned if your physician prefers you remain in a wheelchair until you receive your prosthesis. Most physicians are very conservative with your initial mobility as there is a fall risk with "hopping" on one leg, as well as unnatural stresses on your healthy limb when hopping.

Be prepared to start learning exercises for both your arms and legs to help gain and maintain your strength and range of motion.

Exercise also improves your healing by promoting circulation to your limbs and is well known to help improves mood. The recommended exercises are at the end of this section. Your OT and PT may give you exercises specific to your needs so please perform your prescribed exercise program first, adding the exercises I provide in the book to give yourself additional room and strength.

Discharge from Hospital

As you heal and recover in the hospital, discharge planning will start. Where you go after your hospitalization depends on several key areas. First, there is an evaluation of your home's structure and current setup. Is your home accessible? Is your home a single story or multilevel? Is your bathroom and shower wheelchair accessible?

The second significant factor is whether you live alone or with family/friends. If your home is not wheelchair accessible or you live alone, you may require an extended stay at a skilled nursing facility or acute rehabilitation center. As soon as you are safe in your mobility and are able to perform your activities of daily living, you will be ready to return home.

Return to Home

You have made it home, but the work does not end here. Now is the start of preparing for your future lifestyle. Your rehabilitation actually just begins upon discharge to home, and it is vital you are ready for the work ahead. The next step for many amputees is home health services. This phase of rehabilitation focuses on incision healing (with nurses assisting with dressing changes) and physical therapy for continued strengthening and stretching. Prevention of contractures is essential. If your residual limb becomes tight, losing flexibility and range of motion, this will limit your ability to wear a prosthesis and the ability to walk. I cannot emphasize enough the need to keep your range of motion—contractures will stop you from walking, and they are easy to prevent with proper positioning and exercises.

You will continue to be followed by your surgeon at his office. The time it takes for your incision to heal depends on your health. Your physician will remove your surgical staples/stitches, and once the incision is healed, you will be fitted with a shrinker sock. This sock is a tight elastic sock that is designed to decrease the swelling in your limb and begin shaping it for future prosthetic fitting. Once you are fitted with your shrinker socks, you are ready to start the prosthetic fitting process.

Some patients will be referred to a physician who is a rehabilitation specialist. Physical Medicine and Rehabilitation physicians (also known as physiatrists) have specialized training in amputee rehabilitation. They are an excellent resource for the pre and post-prosthetic fitting phase. They are valuable allies in managing limb sensation and limb pain, and they are able to assist with prosthetic prescriptions and to resolve prosthetic fit issues. If possible, I recommend you find a PM&R physician to work with for your prosthetic needs.

CHAPTER 8

Phantom Limb Sensation and Phantom Limb

Let's take some time to discuss the persistent feeling that you still have your limb. Phantom limb sensation is the perception that an amputated or missing limb is still attached. It is normal and very common for amputees to feel their missing toe itch or sense that their foot is still there. Be cautious at night, as many amputees report falling out of bed because they sense their amputated foot, try to rise out of bed, and soon find themselves on the floor!

Phantom Limb Pain

Phantom limb pain is not a normal sensation. It is different than phantom sensation. The symptoms of phantom pain can be any of these:

- Burning
- Shooting
- "Pins and needles"
- Twisting
- Crushing
- Sensation like an electric shock

Phantom limb pain does have treatment options. Be sure to speak to your physician if you are having any of the above symptoms. Some treatments include:

- Medications
- Compression—wear your compression sock to help
- Massage of the amputation area
- TENS (transcutaneous electrical nerve stimulation) this is a non-invasive technique specific for pain relief
- Heat or cold application
- Biofeedback to reduce muscle tension
- Relaxation techniques
- Injections with local anesthetics and/or steroids
- Nerve blocks
- Surgery to remove scar tissue entangling a nerve

Phantom limb pain can be managed, and wearing a prosthetic limb assists in reducing the painful symptoms. Post-operative pain is different than phantom limb pain and usually decreases as the healing process progresses. Using the techniques above, and improving your mobility with exercise, will decrease the potential for phantom limb pain.

Phantom limb sensation is normal and also decreases with the above pain control suggestions as well as with the fitting of the prosthetic limb. Phantom limb pain is not the norm, but can be successfully managed and may decrease as your rehabilitation process advances. As you increase the time you wear your prosthesis, you may begin to notice a decrease in both phantom pain and phantom sensation as your body adapts to your new socket/prosthetic limb.

CHAPTER 9

Exercises

In this chapter, we are going to talk about some of the most common exercises that are recommended by the physical therapist and the rehab staff. These exercises are chosen based on my years of experience working with patients, but they are listed here as an educational tool and may not be right for you. Make sure to talk to a rehab professional prior to starting any exercises.

Exercises for people with amputations are not just about making sure your muscles are strong. You also need to make sure that you have the right range of motion at the joints around the amputation so that you will be successful with the prosthesis.

These exercises should be started right away, often times starting in the hospital the day after the amputation.

Stretching

First on the list of exercises is stretching. Stretching must be done regularly to maintain the range of motion that our body would normally have.

For example, in the case of an above the knee amputation, the residual limb is often pulled up and flexed toward the front of the body for most of the day including sitting, transfers, and even lying in bed. In order for the prosthesis to properly work the hip needs to be able to extend at least 10 degrees back behind the body.

Another example of an important stretch is for a below the elbow amputee. After the amputation, the body's reaction is to guard the arm and pull it to a bent position near the body. If the elbow and shoulder are not regularly stretched, the arm will become contracted and stuck in that guarded position.

Stretching is by far the most critical exercise for all amputees and needs to be started right away.

The following picture is the most important stretch that can be done for any lower extremity amputee, this position will help to keep the hip extension that will be needed to use any prosthesis correctly in the future.

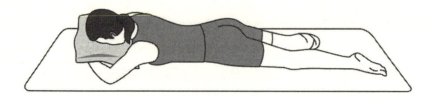

Strengthening

After stretching, you must strengthen the muscles you will need for mobility and prepare the muscles needed for use of the prosthesis.

As you first start to learn how to move with the changes to your body, you will find that you need to be stronger in certain areas to stay safe and mobile. Oftentimes, even the muscles not involved in the amputation area also weaken from the hospital stay and recovery. Below are some common examples of exercises that are critical to a successful recovery.

Examples of common strengthening exercises

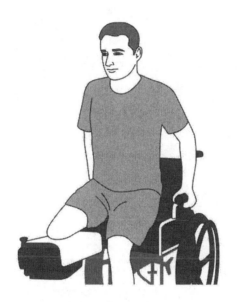

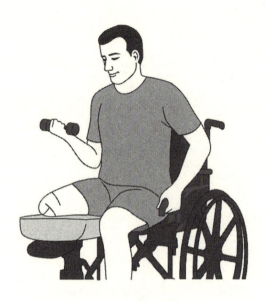
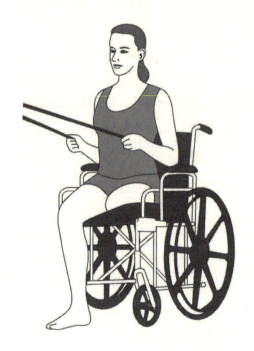

Leg/Lower Extremity Strengthening for Below the Knee Amputations

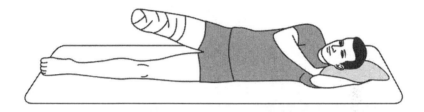

Roll to sound side. Life residual limb straight up and down while keeping hip straight.

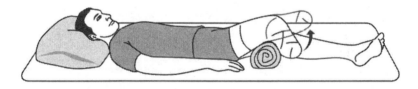

With towel roll behind knee, gently bend and straighten knee over tower roll.

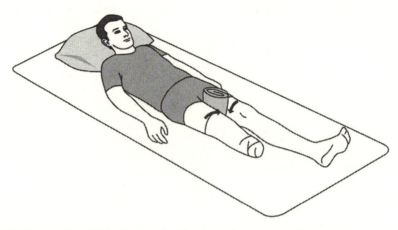

With towel roll between thighs, gently squeeze thighs together and down.

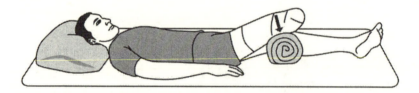

With towel roll under calf of residual limb, tighten thigh muscle to straighten knee. Gently push down while tightening buttock muscles.

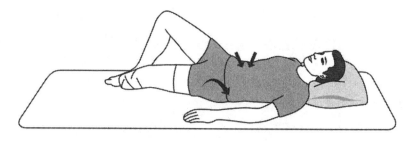

Flatten back by tightening stomach muscles and tilting hips toward waist.

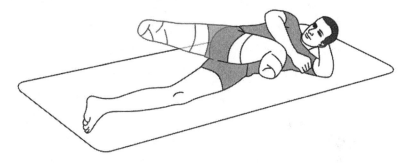

Roll to sound side. Bring knee to chest while bending knee. Reach limb back as far as possible while straightening knee.

Leg/Lower Extremity Strengthening for Above the Knee Amputations

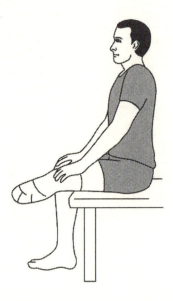

Sitting with residual limb supported, tighten thigh muscle and push down on knee straighten.

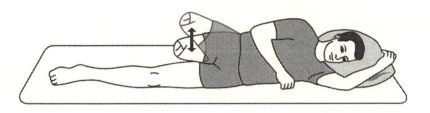

Roll to sound side. Lift residual limb straight up and down while keeping hip straight.

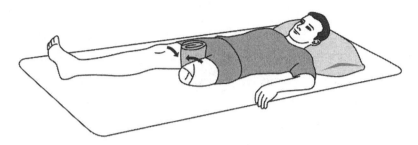

With towel roll between thighs, gently squeeze thighs together and down.

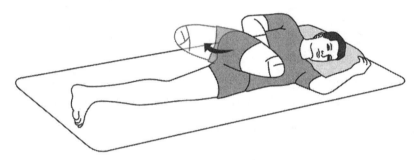

Roll to sound side. Bring residual limb to chest, then reach limb back as far as possible.

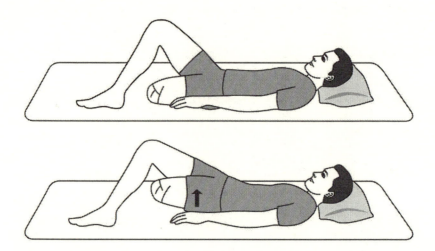

With sound knee bent and foot flat, tighten buttock muscles while attempting to lift hips.

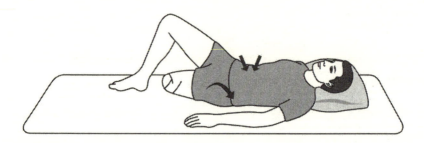

Flatten back by tightening stomach muscles and tilting hips toward waist.

CHAPTER 10

Prosthetic Fitting

Getting a prosthesis that fits well and is able to help you maximize your functional ability is essential for most people with amputations. In this chapter, we are going to discuss some of the things that you need to have in place in order to make that goal a reality.

Before we get back to our amputee stories, let's address the technology information available on the internet. The internet is a *great* source of information, but the technology available in prosthetics does not change the personal journey all amputees have ahead of them.

No matter the tools, learning to walk and learning to return to your activities requires the same muscles, the same balance, and the same (more) endurance than pre-amputation. There is no magic prosthesis that will change your rehabilitation. Explore all your resources on and off the computer, but don't be guided solely by videos from prosthetic companies or their sponsored amputee representatives. Be open to the advice of your peers—like those in this book—and your professional team of therapists, prosthetists, and physicians to find the tools (fancy or not) that will give you the best outcomes for your individual situation.

Understanding Insurance Role with Prosthetic Fitting

The first step in being fitted for a prosthetic limb is initiated by your surgeon or your PM&R physician as a prescription is required by all insurance companies. The prescription must include a K-Level (also known as functional levels). K-Levels are defined by Medicare based on an individual's ability or potential to ambulate and navigate their environment. Once your K-Level has been determined by the physician for an individual, the doctor can then determine which prosthetic components are covered by Medicare and other insurance. It is important to re-emphasize that a medical doctor (treating physician) must make this determination.

What this means is simply that your K-Level directs what type of foot/ankle, knee joint, hip joint, and socket suspension system your prosthetist is able to choose from.

The different K-Levels are:

Level 0: Does not have the ability or potential to ambulate or transfer safely with or without assistance and a prosthetic limb does not enhance their quality of life or mobility.

Level 1: Has the ability or potential to use a prosthetic limb for transfers or ambulation on level surfaces at fixed cadence. Common for the amputee with limited and unlimited household ambulation.

Level 2: Has the ability or potential for ambulation with the ability to traverse low-level environmental barriers such as curbs, stairs or uneven surfaces. Commonly labeled limited community ambulator.

Level 3: Has the ability or potential for ambulation with variable cadence. Common of the community ambulator who has the ability to traverse most environmental barriers and may have vocational, therapeutic, or exercise activity that demands prosthetic utilization beyond simple locomotion.

Level 4: Has the ability or potential for prosthetic ambulation that exceeds basic ambulation skills, exhibiting high impact, stress, or energy levels. This group has the prosthetic demands of a child, active adult, or athlete.

After receiving your prescription for your prosthetic limb, the next step is selecting a prosthetist. Selecting a prosthetist is a very important task. Your prosthetist follows you for the remainder of your life, continually working with you to replace your prosthetic limb as needed. At the start of the fitting process, the prosthetist should take measurements of your limb to follow the changing shape and loss of fluid (edema). Waiting for the swelling to decrease gives you a better fitting socket (the part of the prosthesis that your residual limb sits in).

Initiation of Prosthetic fitting

The prosthetic fitting process takes several weeks to complete. Once the amputated limb has stabilized in volume, the prosthetist will make a cast of the limb. The cast is used to make a "test" socket. The test socket is a clear plastic that assists the prosthetist in fitting the socket specifically to your limb shape. If the fit is correct, the test socket is finished with a sturdy laminate cover. You will likely have weekly visits to the prosthetist during the fitting process. Once the prosthetic limb is delivered, you will continue to see the prosthetist for alignment and socket adjustments, although this will not be as frequent as the fitting stages. Your first prosthetic limb is called the "preparatory" prosthesis, as this initial fit is very likely to change as you continue to improve your mobility and lose volume in your amputated limb. The time in your preparatory prosthesis is very individualized with some patients requiring re-socketing more than once, while others may stay in their preparatory prosthesis for a year or more.

You will continue to lose volume (or shrink) with your initial socket, and this is normal. Patients can go through multiple sockets if they continue to shrink, and others will have the original socket for many years as their leg fluid volume does not change as dramatically. The prosthetist will educate you and provide prosthetic socks, which are necessary for every amputee to learn how to use. Using the prosthetic socks is the most important skill to learn as a new amputee. The continued fit of your prosthetic socket can only be maintained by adjusting the sock ply you are wearing. It is a daily and continuous challenge to maintain the socket fit. Poor prosthetic sock management can lead to unwanted complications—the worst being blistering on your limb making you unable able to wear your prosthetic limb.

Learning how to use your prosthetic limb

Outpatient physical therapy will start once you receive your preparatory prosthesis. Outpatient therapy is usually not required pre-prosthetic fitting as the patient should have received exercises for strengthening and stretching and education in preventing contractures during their hospitalization and again with home health.

A severely deconditioned patient will benefit from outpatient therapy to improve their endurance/strength and stretch out any contractures. However, it is essential for physical therapy or occupational therapy to start once the patient receives their prosthesis. Outpatient therapy will work on teaching the patient how to use their new artificial limb including how to use prosthetic socks to manage their prosthetic socket fit properly. The therapist will reinforce the proper donning/doffing of a prosthesis, skin care (essential for all amputees), and focus on safe technique with emphasis on the patient achieving their most functional independence with their prosthetic device. This includes gait training with the lower extremity amputee and hand training for the upper extremity amputee. Again, the primary focus of these therapies is to assist each patient to reach their highest level of independence.

New amputees need to be realistic about their unique challenges. The energy required to walk with a prosthetic limb is well documented. The higher the level of amputation, the more caloric energy expenditure is required to walk. The requirements are as follows:

- Single Below the knee amputee requires 30% more caloric expenditure to walk
- Double below the knee amputee requires 40% more caloric expenditure to walk
- Single Above the knee amputee requires 65-80% more caloric expenditure to walk—dependent on patient's vascular condition
- Double above the knee amputee requires 110% more energy to walk

Depending on a patient's health, it may not be best for a patient to walk for all activities. Amputees may need to accept their physical limitations for walking and conserve their energy for other activities by continuing to use a wheelchair. Balancing your lifestyle and activities for your level of physical fitness is very important. Some amputees will require walkers, crutches, or canes to walk. Reaching your safest most independent lifestyle is the goal, and there should be no judgment on what devices help you reach your goals. Please note, the energy levels required to walk do not change based on your prosthetic device. To date, there is no prosthesis that does the walking for you. Thus the muscle energy required is the same no matter what type of prosthesis you have.

May I also reiterate that technological information available on the internet may, or may not, help. I acknowledge that the internet is a *great* source of information, but I strongly encourage the readers of this book to understand that the technology available in prosthetics does not change the personal journey all amputees have ahead of them. At the start of this chapter, I stated that the post-operative rehabilitation through the pre-prosthetic fitting is very standardized and only varies by length of time each patient spends in each of these early phases.

Carol: Quadrilateral Amputee with Bilateral Below the Knee and Bilateral Below the Elbow Amputations Due to Sepsis

Carol's rehabilitation was very different from the norm. She had lost all four limbs, and she was expected to have a long rehabilitation recovery period. Carol was deemed medically stable while in the trauma unit after her surgeries, and she was discharged to a skilled nursing facility on a long-term rehabilitation plan. During her stay, she developed a bladder infection and became seriously ill so she was transferred back to the hospital for medical care.

As Carol recovered from this setback, she was accepted into the acute rehabilitation unit at the hospital. She began a four-month stay starting with three hours per day of physical therapy and occupational therapy. Carol began her prosthetic rehabilitation while in the acute care unit. She was fitted for her lower extremity prosthetic limbs during her stay and she continued her extensive physical and occupational therapy—learning how to transfer and walk with a specialized walker.

Carol remembers the overwhelming joy she experienced with her first walk in her new prosthetic limbs. That was the moment she knew that her future was going to be okay. Her progress was slow but steady. As her walking progressed, she moved to the next step of being fitted for her upper extremity prostheses. She was again unusually fitted with her body-powered "hook" (prosthetic limb) in the hospital. Continued therapy in the hospital prepared Carol for her return home.

Carol's family built a ramp and remodeled her bathroom so she would have wheelchair access to everything. Remember, you may not always be wearing your prosthetic limbs into your bathroom, especially for showering, and you will need to have an accessible bathroom to be able to return home. One special feature of Carol's bathroom remodel was the purchase of a Toto Japanese toilet. This style of toilet is extremely helpful as Carol's prosthetic limbs would not be functional for toiletry skills. She encourages all quadrilateral amputees to look at this option to maximize their independence.

Completing her inpatient rehabilitation for Carol was only a first step. She transitioned to outpatient physical therapy and occupational therapy. As her skills improved, she was eligible for new arm prosthetics and was fitted for myoelectric prostheses. Carol remarks that these prostheses are more comfortable than the body-powered prostheses with the straps, but she soon discovered the use of universal attachments, which became her most functional tools for bathing, dressing, and eating.

Carol achieved her goals. She now starts her mornings by donning her prosthetic legs when she wakes up. She uses multiple prosthetic "tools" for her arms to do her tasks independently. She walks without any assistive device and walks daily for exercise around her ranch. Truly inspirational!

Ray: Right Hip Disarticulation Due to Cancer

Ray was excited to move forward and anxious to get walking. Ray had been inactive for a long time and his weight increased to about 250 lbs. His initial prosthetic limb fitting took eight months. Between waiting and not having a hip, Ray truly began to believe Dr. Shin was wrong. He was getting depressed and thought there wasn't going to be a prosthesis for him, thinking that walking was just a dream.

Eventually, Ray received word from the prosthetic company that the fitting process could begin, but it still took several more months before he received his first prosthesis. Finally, Ray was ready to learn to walk.

However, it just wasn't happening for him; Ray wasn't able to walk. He was working with physical therapy but wasn't making much progress, and he became convinced it was his fault. What was he doing wrong? Was he stupid? Why couldn't he get this prosthesis to work? He went back to the prosthetist who told him "you are fat, and that is the problem." He also informed Ray that Medicare would never give him another hip—this is all he got.

Ray was distraught, discouraged, and downhearted. He couldn't walk without falling. Ray didn't want to hear false praise; he wanted the truth.

Ray decided to seek a consultation with another prosthetist. The new prosthetist frankly told Ray—this is not your fault. The hip joint is not a good choice for you as the hip joint and knee joint don't match, and the socket doesn't fit correctly. It was all wrong.

Ray felt hope—just maybe he would walk again.

The first prosthesis was a nightmare; the parts didn't work for Ray. The parts he needed had to be just right because he has a hip disarticulation. Ray received a new socket and new components and for the first time, his prosthesis felt like a part of him. Ray began walking, at first with a walker and then with crutches. His wheelchair was stored in the back of his truck—where it remains today.

Ray continued to lose weight; the weight loss was purposeful. Ray wanted to protect his right knee (which had severe degenerative joint disease), lower his cholesterol (which he did), and increase his energy (which has hugely improved). He is currently down to 175 pounds. Ray has had several new sockets made, and recently a new hip/knee joint combination and a new foot with an articulating ankle. Ray's gait is so much easier, and he is living his life in the foothills of California with excitement and *great* anticipation of more prosthetic inventions to improve his walking even more.

Larry: Bilateral Below the Knee Amputee Due to diabetes

It took 10 months before Larry received his first prosthesis due to slow healing of his right leg. He feels that physical therapy was key as it taught him not only how to walk, but also how to balance and how to use stairs and ramps. He was pleased with his progress and was feeling blessed.

After a while, Larry's other foot experienced the same issue as his right, and he had to undergo a second amputation. His second amputation was 1.5 years after the first. Larry matter-of-factly planned on getting the second prosthetic limb to walk. His left leg healed in 6 months and Larry received his left prosthesis shortly after.

Larry, like Ray, always knew he was going to be okay. Larry did everything he was instructed to do. He practiced his exercises, he practiced his walking on his ramp, and he felt himself getting stronger.

Motivation was never an issue and Larry didn't meet any other amputees. He is very independent and has to do things for himself.

His greatest motivation is his wife. He prayed every time he was seated in his car that he would not need his wife to lift, load, and unload his wheelchair from the trunk of the car. Larry was determined, and certain he was going to walk.

After therapy was completed, Larry knew he no longer needed his wheelchair, and he felt he had made it. Larry had made a promise to help his wife, and he feels very blessed to this day that he was able to reach his goals and keep that promise.

Jon: Right Knee Disarticulation Due to Trauma

Jon's rehabilitation was different from the others mentioned in this book as he suffered multiple traumas from his accident. In addition to the artery issue, He also incurred an ACL tear, MCL sprain, and a tibial plateau fracture. Jon was discharged in a wheelchair but was very fired up to start his rehab. Jon perceived every transition as positive, and every new progress propelled him forward in his rehab. He remembers getting so excited about his evolution from being totally dependent in the hospital and then slowly gaining his independence in a wheelchair, then getting sick of his wheelchair and going to crutches. He then went from loving his crutches to hating his crutches to wanting a cane. After getting a cane, he was determined to get rid of it completely. After he accomplished that, he turned his goals toward running and then wanting to do marathons. Always having a next goal was his therapy while also admitting his impatience with his current situation. Jon always wanted to be at the next level. As he achieved his goals, he would then reset for the next level of goals. The hardest stage for someone like Jon is when all the goals are over—then what?

Jon's first PM&R physician through his workers comp was from a different medical institution, not UCD Health. Working with this particular physician was the only negative experience of all of Jon's rehabilitation process. Jon was frustrated, and his physician was unwilling to take advice from experts. Jon knew it wasn't a match and switched.

He says it was a natural transition to attend outpatient PT due to the department already being a part of UCD Health. Jon was referred to the PM&R Amputee Clinic where he was introduced to the prosthetists and his prosthetic team. Jon doesn't remember having a choice but instantly feeling comfortable with Ann Theabold, CPO from Hanger. All of the members of Jon's team were fired up to work with him. His energy was so positive that everyone working with him seemed to feed off of it. The team always worked on being perfect, and this was a huge motivator for Jon. He was compliant and listened to all the instructions and understood why those instructions were so important to perform and it worked. And it was awesome. The message of working on being perfect was the same as Jon's philosophy.

His current employer was holding his job for him, but Jon was not going to be able to return to work as he could no longer climb poles. The obvious "unables" were easy for him to swallow. It was the close "almosts" that were hard for him to take, and someone saying "you can't" was not acceptable to Jon.

Regardless, Jon needed to get back to work. So he contacted his new company while on crutches, and they were encouraging. The company told him to get his prosthesis, and they would have a job for him when he came back. Six months after his amputation, Jon returned to work in a transition position. Jon was feeling pretty good and staying very busy with work and his many medical appointments.

While Jon was attending physical therapy for his left leg injuries, he read an article about Sarah Rhinehart, an above the knee amputee who had just finished competing and completing the

Ironman competition. Jon says he didn't connect to it at first. Jon's shift into athletics actually started with golf. He learned about the adaptive golf program offered at Haggin Oaks Golf Course. Jon took private lessons, and as with all his rehab, Jon was there to learn the "perfect" swing. The idea of "perfect" is Jon's motto for taking on challenges, and as he worked with his instructor, Jon became very involved in the sport of golf.

Playing golf then evolved to Jon's desire to try running. Jon admits he is very lucky that he had insurance, which covered the cost of his sports prosthetics. He went through the approval process and received the type of prosthesis he needed to run. The first thought was to have a running leg that he could also walk with, but that didn't work. Jon and his prosthetist realized a prosthesis designed for multiple tasks performed poorly for both tasks. If you want to run, especially competitive running, you will need a separate running prosthesis. Jon ran his first 5K in November, just 10 months after his amputation. But the prosthesis was heavy and forced an unnatural gait with running. So Jon upgraded to a flex foot and his running took off. He was receiving *great*, positive feedback from his family, friends, coworkers, and his medical team and that energy just gave him more fuel to keep setting more goals. So Jon reached out to Challenged Athletes Foundation and entered an aquathon, which is a swim/run combination. Jon was hooked, and his next 2–3 years he became completely dedicated to triathlons.

Jon was doing well with his triathlons when a friend invited him to try mountain biking. Biking became Jon's next challenge, and he began competing in mountain biking triathlons becoming the first above knee amputee to complete a full Xterra Triathlon. Jon still recalls this being the hardest race he has ever done. He had to learn how to open water swim, learn how to run, and learn how to ride both road and mountain bikes.

So what was next? Jon recognized how supportive his family (specifically his wife) was with his need for athletics. His wife understood that participation in sports was a part of Jon's therapy. Between working full time and the amount of training time required to compete, Jon was ready to transition to other sports and spend more time with his family. Jon moved into CrossFit for 2 years and then did a stint with Jiu-Jitsu for several months.

Megan: Below the Knee Amputation Due to Congenital Abnormality
Megan had little rehabilitation. Being a teenager with limited mobility with her left foot for years, she was ready to be a normal kid. She only required a few sessions of physical therapy to learn how to strengthen her left leg and understand what normal gait was. She was off and moving with no looking back.

Prosthetically, however, Megan's first prosthesis was all about the "skin" or covering. As a young woman, she was only interested in appearance and not in functionality. As she has matured, she naturally moved toward the importance of functionality over appearance. Unbeknownst to Megan at the time, was the battle she would have with her insurance company. As stated, amputees will "shrink out" of their preparatory prosthetic socket and require new sockets to be made. Megan's insurance denied her socket replacement stating it was not a medical necessity. She was wearing an 18-ply thickness of sock and was challenged to walk. After going through the appeal process, the insurance company agreed to pay for the new socket. She has learned that what you see on the internet—all the fancy skins and "higher end" prosthetic devices are not covered by insurances and also do not contribute to your functional level, which is most important over time.

Jake: Bilateral Below the Knee Amputations Due to Trauma
Jake chose not to go to an acute rehabilitation program. He asked what he would learn in rehab, and when he was told that he would

learn self-care activities, he chose to practice these skills while in the hospital to see if he could learn them on his own. Jake was anxious to get home and wanted to learn these activities of daily living without transferring to rehab, which would lead to a more extensive hospital stay. He began learning transfers from his bed to a wheelchair and was able to learn different self-care techniques for his activities of daily living—toiletry, bathing, and dressing until he mastered each skill so he could return home. Each challenge was a goal to get him to the next step.

Jake started outpatient physical therapy for pre-prosthetic training and exercise, and this again established challenges and goals for Jake to work toward. His constant motivation was the goals of returning to work, returning to his family in the States, and returning to his family at the South Pole.

As each goal for independence was met at the wheelchair level, Jake became fixated on his goal of walking again. Jake had no expectations with prosthetics. He recalls his best experience in the hospital was meeting another triple amputee who had above the knee and the elbow amputations. Jake remembers this amputee challenging him to be better since he had knees and elbows. Jake's fitting process, again was unique to his situation. For Jake, the fitting process began with his right arm prosthesis. He was fitted with his right upper extremity prosthesis and began occupational therapy to learn how to use a prosthesis always, always, keeping his determination at the forefront of reaching his ultimate goal—complete independence.

Jake feels fortunate that he was able to initiate his right arm prosthetic while in the hospital and start OT with his right prosthesis before he started the fitting phase of his lower extremities. Being able to work on one body part's rehabilitation permitted Jake a focus point and the ability to set up his rehab goals in a progressive manner. He also began recovering use of his left fingers as his healing process continued. Jake was determined that his right arm prosthesis be as functional, if not more, than his left hand. With his rehabilitation, Jake stayed so focused and motivated that he even learned to write with his right-hand prosthetic limb!

Jake was discharged to his parents' home and continued rehabilitating his arms/hands as an outpatient. Then the next phase of fitting his lower leg prostheses began. The upper extremity prosthesis is non-weight bearing, which is very different than lower leg prosthetic limbs. The fitting of the upper arm socket is important but not as important as the socket fit of the leg prosthesis. There are a lot of body changes during the fitting process, with the leg shrinking and losing volume. Jake was one of the patients that required multiple sockets to be made during his fitting process. Jake just kept listening to his prosthetist and his physical therapist, and he reports that understanding the process was very helpful—keeping him on track to reaching his goals.

Carlos: Right Above the Knee Amputation Due to Arteriosclerosis and Blood Clots

Carlos spent two weeks in the hospital and was then discharged home in a wheelchair. He had to take the time for both his left and right legs to heal. He received home health services for dressing changes and exercise. Carlos had his stitches removed approximately seven weeks after his surgery. Two to three weeks later, he was cleared by his surgeon to start his fitting for his preparatory prosthesis. Carlos received a list of prosthetic companies for him to contact, and he chose the prosthetic company closest to his home. He was also referred to UCD Health PM&R Amputee Clinic and Dr. Shin.

Carlos was ready to start his prosthetic rehabilitation. His preparatory prosthesis had a hydraulic, mechanical knee. He completed a course of physical therapy and was independently walking. Carlos walked everywhere and was not using any assistive device. The more he walked, the more he fell, a total of 32 falls in one and a half years! Yes, he counted every fall. Carlos returned to his prosthetist and through his military VA benefits was able to "upgrade" his definitive prosthesis to a microprocessor knee. Carlos has never had another fall after finding the right prosthetic componentry for his level of activity.

Carlos understood the process: the patient must demonstrate their skill and activity level with a mechanical knee before insurances will pay for a more complex, expensive microprocessor knee. He understood his responsibility as a walker to demonstrate and work to the skill level required to advance his knee component. Carlos also understood that all amputees have different health conditions that impact their ability to walk. He challenges all amputees to push themselves to reach their highest skill level, and maximize their functional levels. He has always been happy with his rehab journey as each challenge he faced brought greater gains to his independence.

The rehabilitative phase starts as soon as your surgery is completed and continues until you reach your full potential. It includes a medical team that is there to push you and support you during this phase of your recovery. The responsibility though lies squarely on the patient. Perform your exercises, listen and comply with your instructions, and do not use the internet as your primary source of information. The rehabilitation phase is not easy, and it is okay to remind yourself of the constant forward/backward stages, which are all natural with amputee rehabilitation. The work is worth it. With your commitment, working with your team, and a willingness to challenge yourself, you can successfully reach your goals and rehab potential.

PART IV

Moving Forward/Acceptance

CHAPTER 11

Physical needs

At the time of your discharge to home, hopefully, the adaptive equipment has been obtained, and your home is set up for your return. Home modifications are not always able to be completed before your discharge. It is fine to be home and assist in learning what adaptations and modifications work best for your needs. Do you need a ramp to get into your home? Is your bathroom accessible for a wheelchair? Or will a bedside commode be a temporary solution? Is your shower a walk-in style or a tub/shower combination? Do you need a tub bench or shower chair? Grab bars are considered a must in the shower and by your toilet, and are inexpensive and easy to install. Another suggestion is to be sure a handrail is installed next to any stairway that has more than two steps.

For upper extremity amputees with concerns about independent toileting, technology has improved and toilets are on the market that can assist with self-cleaning, push-button flushing, and other amenities. Who knew? This is an example of how talking with other amputees could give you the information that will provide you the utmost independence in your own home!

The initial prosthetic limb you receive is called a "preparatory" limb. In more detail, the preparatory limb is your first socket. Depending on your diagnosis, healing process, and activity level you may need replacement sockets to maintain a good prosthetic fit, or you may remain in the initial socket for a long time. A good fitting socket is the primary need of an amputee to ambulate. It does not matter whether it is the original socket or several replacement sockets. Once your limb has stabilized in volume size, your socket will become your "definitive" prosthesis. A definitive prosthesis is considered your finished prosthesis, which includes your individualized componentry. Componentry refers to the type of foot, or knee joint on your prosthetic limb.

You will still be followed closely by your prosthetist. Your limb may potentially change, and socket adjustments will need to be completed. Your alignment may require fine tuning as you begin to ambulate more frequently or over longer distances. The life of a prosthesis averages five years, depending again on your activity level.

This is a special note for amputees with higher-level amputations as there is often an extra step required by insurance companies before you receive your definitive prosthetic limb. The newest technology is amazing, but as previously mentioned, not appropriate for all amputees. And new technology is extremely expensive. Insurance companies, rightfully so, do not want to pay for technology that will not be used by the patient. It is an acceptable practice to have the amputee's preparatory, prosthetic limb be solely functional using traditional componentry to learn how to walk. As the patient improves his or her skill level and K-Level, there will be video or documentation provided to request authorization for the higher, technological components. Please remember, technology does not "walk" by itself; the patient must provide all the energy and muscle movement to ambulate. If you are not able to ambulate with traditional joints, you will not be able to walk with a "computerized" knee.

So what is the advantage of a computer knee? There is one significant advantage of a microprocessor knee, and it is called stumble recovery. The computer will recognize certain missteps, which permits users a brief moment to catch themselves from falling. The knee will stiffen as it identifies the misstep allowing the patients to stabilize themselves. Stumble recovery is a great tool and will require some additional training to learn to use correctly. If you feel you are a candidate for the microprocessor knee you must be open to a very frank discussion with your prosthetic team on the pros/cons of your specific case.

For upper extremity prosthetics, computerized technology is more complicated. The traditional body-powered elbow or shoulder joint is still the most functional of all prosthetic limbs. The attachments that are available provide the most flexibility in being independent with your daily activities. Myoelectric prosthetic limbs have specific benefits as well as challenges. And the new technology being developed for fingers/hands is promising, but as to the date of this book it is still limited in functional uses. The exciting future of prosthetics will bring so many advancements, but today, please stay focused on which technology will provide you the greatest functional independence.

The definitive, prosthetic limb will likely need replacement every three to five years. The process of making the new device will be the same as the process of making your preparatory prosthesis with the added opportunity to discuss any changes in your functional level with your prosthetist. The prosthetist will work with you on updating your components to fit your lifestyle needs, to help you maintain your highest level of independence, and to update you on changing technology when you are being fitted for your next definitive, prosthetic limb. The future of prosthetics is unpredictable and exciting! Your team will be able to help you come up with the best prosthetic limb for you. Remember that it is a very individual prescription.

CHAPTER 12

Emotional needs

Stages of emotional recovery are different from the physical recovery stages. With physical recovery, it is more of a check off list as you succeed at each new step. Occasionally, there are back steps such as the development of a rash or waiting for your prosthesis to be re-adjusted, but there is always forward progress.

With emotional recovery, patients and families may move back and forth between the stages of grief. Moving between stages is normal. As you physically improve, your emotional challenges may fluctuate. Remember, there is no one way to emotionally heal. The path toward acceptance is individualistic, but as a reminder, you are not the only person to travel the emotional healing road. The recommendations on emotional recovery from the previous chapter provide the same practical tools for your post-rehabilitation phase of emotional recovery. Seek out other amputees, support groups, books, or counseling, and do your best to keep open communication with your family/caregivers about your feelings, no matter how frequently your feelings change.

There is one significant change I recommend to improve your emotional well-being and to move forward toward acceptance. **Wear your prosthesis!** The impact of wearing your prosthesis is huge. Your prosthesis should be donned first thing in the morning, and be the last item doffed in the evening. By wearing your prosthesis regularly, your body's neurological system begins to make sensory adjustments and will accept your prosthesis physically as a part of your body. As your physical body accepts your new limb, your emotional state will catch up. The best walkers and users of prosthetic limbs are the people who use their devices daily. When a patient is struggling with learning to use their new prosthetic limb, I always ask how much they wear it. And the answer is always, "Sometimes." Wear your prosthesis, even when not going out or not walking. If you are not physically wearing your prosthetic limb, the acceptance phase is nearly impossible to achieve.

CHAPTER 13

Advice from Our Amputees

Learning from those that have gone before is always valuable. The amputees interviewed in this book wish to share their experiences, wisdom, and advice to pave an easier journey for all new amputees and their families. Here is what they have to say:

Carol: Quadrilateral Amputee with Bilateral Below Knee and Bilateral Below Elbow Amputations Due to Sepsis
Carol's advice: "No doubt some of you have had your challenges and have learned your own way of coping. Here are a few of my thoughts. It is very important to get started and take that first step forward to give life a chance even though a person might not be in the mood for it. It is not a new idea to find your strengths through adversity and to learn things about yourself and others. I am very aware now of basic human goodness. People really do want to help and ease suffering when it is present.

We all want to remain independent. I do most stuff for myself just fine, but obviously, I do need help in some areas. I have learned to trust people and will ask for help if I need it. Friend or stranger, there has never been a refusal. Some just know and jump in, but for others, there might be a little shyness even about approaching. I find that it is good to be welcoming and let them know that I am appreciative that they care. Everyone faces challenges in life, and maybe that person is dealing with difficulty themselves. The upside is that it gets us thinking outward and away from ourselves.

So surround yourself with good people. Be welcoming and respectful to others—let them lift your spirits. Good people will do just that.

I accept almost all invitations. At first, I was reluctant to go out socially, but my husband wasn't having any of that, and I soon found that going out was still very fun. I can't get enough of that now.

I look for things to be thankful for. Besides blessings that I have mentioned, I live in a time where amazing technological advances help me function way beyond what I might have imagined even eight years ago (hands for example).

There is always humor—look for laughter. Look for the ridiculous—it is everywhere, even in a hospital. For example, on a return check up to see the amputee doctor, the nurse who knew my story had me stand on the scale for the required weigh-in, looking down she admired my shoes and said, "Are they comfortable?" Actually, along with being funny, it was a nice moment because she had forgotten all about the disability and that is always neat.

So when times are tough, push yourself to give life a chance. For me, it was worth it. That is pretty much the story. I am flattered to be considered resilient."

Larry: Bilateral Below the Knee Amputee Due to diabetes

Larry is now 80 years old and says he has slowed down, but he isn't stopping. Larry doesn't notice a difference between having one or two prosthetic limbs. "I knew how to deal with one, now I just deal with two, and it isn't different." His general attitude is, "Hey, it could be worse." Larry is always thankful for all the things he can do—he is independent with his activities, he can go out and water his yard, and he cooks and loves his family barbeques.

Larry's advice, "Do not give up. If you feel you can do it, you can. You can do a lot of things if you think you can. You may have to figure out a different way and you may fail a few times until you figure it out, but don't quit. If you think you can't, you won't."

Larry does have a secret that he used to accomplish some of his goals. He always waited for his wife to go to church and while he was alone, he would take the time to go figure out how to do certain things. One challenge Larry took head on—trying to drive. While his wife was putting away the groceries, Larry backed the car out and drove around the block. He pulled back into the driveway and told his wife that he realized he was going to have to give up driving. He knew he had no feeling in his legs and it just wasn't safe, but he had to try. Larry's wife doesn't mind driving, and Larry says he has the most beautiful chauffeur in the world.

To this day he still feels very blessed, and he thanks the Good Lord for being there and for getting him to where he is now. "I may not be all the way back, but I am close."

Ray: Right Hip Disarticulation Due to Cancer

Ray is down to 175 pounds. Ray has had several new sockets made and recently a new hip/knee joint combination with a new foot with an articulating ankle. Ray's gait is so much easier now, and he is living his life in the foothills of California with excitement and *great* anticipation of more prosthetic inventions to keep improving his walking.

Ray feels there is more to do with his life. He confesses, he doesn't know what it is or what it will be, but he was never, ever ready to die. Ray is not angry. He asks "why be mad? NOOO!" He outlived all the predictions of his demise! That alone is a reason to be happy and to live.

From day one of his amputation to date, Ray's life is a million times greater than he ever anticipated. He does everything he wants and needs to do. His future is bright.

Ray's inspiration is everything that all the doctors/therapists have done to get him to where he is today. He admits he had hard times, but he never wavered—giving up is never an option when you have so many folks working to help you get better, you get inspired to get better. "The people who had faith and belief in me, that was my inspiration, and I could not let them down."

His pastor calls Ray a street evangelist—he walks his dog daily and talks to people and tells his story. Ray doesn't feel he is an inspiration to others and is uncomfortable with those labels. Ray encourages everyone to move forward, "Don't give up and don't let people down." And Ray is very excited to be a part of this book. When he had his amputation, Ray searched all over the internet for information regarding hip disarticulation. He couldn't find anyone to meet or talk to regarding his amputation. He is ready to share his story to help other amputees, particularly those with hip disarticulations. Ray is very hopeful about all the opportunities ahead. After all, dying is still not scheduled in his day planner.

Jon: Right Knee Disarticulation Due to Trauma

Now at age 43, Jon is more focused on family and work. With his left leg developing arthritis and the higher risk of falls/injury with his high-intensity training and also with his children being older, Jon has moved away from athletics. He is grateful his work was so supportive of his sports activities, and now he is working at a hard job and is succeeding. His journey is changing to focus on reaching his retirement age of 55 and focus on getting his children to college. He still has hobbies and is very active in woodworking. And he has become more safety conscious—partly due to his work, but more importantly as part of securing a better future.

Jon does admit to feeling a slight void without exercise, but he is okay with that. Jon gives himself credit for his accomplishments, but he doesn't feel it does any good to believe your life is harder than someone else's. The reality is that the world doesn't care. We all have to get up each day, do our best, and pay the bills. Life becomes more normal, and like most of us, every morning he still wakes up wishing he could shut off the alarm and sleep more, but he gets up and puts his leg on and moves into his day.

Advice is difficult to give as it is dependent on the individual. Jon does recommend to all amputees to be engaged with their rehab, which will engage the team, and help set and reach your goals. He feels blessed he has a good prosthetist and warns others that prosthetic limbs are a business and to be wary in a difficult world to traverse. There are new amputees struggling to get back on track working with companies that will make money off of them. It is a concern and patients need to be aware of the conflict—needing to be sure to be with someone who has their best interest. There is a 3-5 year commitment to wearing your prosthesis, so a good fit and the right componentry is essential or you can end up with a useless prosthesis. Jon is grateful he often has the opportunity to trial new products and works closely with his prosthetist to evaluate the benefits and pitfalls of new technology in prosthetic devices as they emerge.

Athletics is challenging. As with all athletes, you must be willing to take the risk of injury and likely falls, and you must be willing to ask for help. Jon tells the story, "I was training for a triathlon. During a training run, I ran up onto a curb and my prosthesis broke right at a busy intersection. The knee joint completely fell off. Luckily a passerby gave me a ride home."

Megan: Below the Knee Amputation Due to Congenital Abnormality
Megan is now 28 years old, married, and expecting her first child. She says the differences between men and women and prosthetics is very compelling. She better understands that her appearance is no longer her primary concern, but being able to function is the priority. Her advice for new amputees is to learn realistic expectations. She firmly believes being an amputee is not very limiting. Amputees have to grasp that their life is theirs to live. Being an amputee just means you may have to do things differently.

Carlos: Above the Knee Amputation Due to Arteriosclerosis and Blood Clots
Carlos started working with children with special needs during his high school years. Becoming an amputee didn't change his mindset of giving back to the community, but now as an amputee, he changed his target audience. He became an amputee peer counselor for new amputees. Carlos took training classes to become a certified peer counselor and he gets calls from the local hospitals to visit new amputees to provide support and to educate the new patient in their future endeavors. He goes to patients' homes and helps train them in transfers and setting up their homes for improved functionality.

Carlos was invited to attend an amputee support group in his area. There were only five people in the group. He attended a few more sessions and decided to not only embrace this group, but to activate it by developing the idea of starting a nonprofit organization to support amputees. Out of this, Gold Country Amputee Support Group was founded. The group has now grown to 50 members and meets twice a month.

Carlos says, "There is life after amputation. Why give up?" He continues to challenge himself as well; Carlos is about to join an amputee dance group and challenge himself to learn how to dance.

Jake: Bilateral Below the Knee Amputations Due to Trauma

Jake was 39 and had been married for two years at the time of his accident. Now Jake marks the anniversary date May 22, 2009 as the start of his new life. Jake and his wife have moved back to New Zealand to a small farm near a town with a population of around 550 people.

Jake prefers using his body-powered arm prosthesis as he is very hard on his prosthesis. He does have a myoelectric prosthetic limb, but for Jake, the myoelectric type breaks easily and is very restrictive in its uses. He reports he uses his "hook" 90% of the time and only uses his myoelectric prosthesis 10 % of the time, more for social events. Living out in the country, and farming, and being 600 miles away from the nearest prosthetist, Jake has taught himself how to be creative, and how to problem solve at getting his work done. Jake has developed his own terminal devices to use as tools for his work. He feels the toolkit helps him with functionality. Jake says it will take trial and errors to succeed, but always keep practicing and working toward perfection. When you find what works for you keep working on the fine-tuning.

Jake believes the future of prosthetic limbs needs to be in the direction of versatility, flexibility, and durability. For Jake, his prostheses were all about functionality—from cooking dinner to setting up scientific gear. Prosthetics is very personal and individualistic, but he says no technology is as important as the need for a *great* fitting socket. If the socket isn't correct, no technology can help you function better.

Jake strongly believes amputees should recognize that being an amputee may not be the cause of changes in your life, but may just be a part of growing and the normal life changes that come with aging. There is life after amputation and people do lead healthy, active lives. Jake advises to meet new amputees at the hospital and be welcoming to the newest member of the club. He acknowledges that the mental part is the hardest. Jake learned to admit that it hurt. It is difficult, but learning to ask for help and then not being angry that you asked for help is a valuable skill for amputees. He encourages new amputees to gauge frustration levels and work on communication skills. Sometimes letting people help you is more about helping them feel better about themselves versus you actually needing the help. Work on being inclusive and always appreciate those trying to help you.

Jake is very comfortable with who he is. His philosophy: "I don't believe being amputated changes your whole personality of who you were, you retain a majority of your original personality, and you then figure out how to put these new bits into your personality—the person you are now."

Conclusion

There is hope, happiness, and full, meaningful lives after limb loss. Remember, amputation is ultimately the treatment of choice for saving your life and is performed due to medical necessity. Not only does this treatment save your life, but amputation of a limb enables you to resume your independent lifestyle and retain being an active member of society. Loss of a limb is very similar to loss of a loved one in terms of grieving, and although difficult, we do move forward with our lives.

The goal of this book was to help others learn and understand the medical reasons for amputation and to be educated in the rehabilitation process. Knowledge does lead to an easier transition for patients and families to move into their post-limb amputation lives. Being prepared for the physical changes and more importantly the emotional stages will decrease the stress of the "unknown." Providing resources will also help steer you through your rehabilitation process. I hope this book helps all who read it to regain their independence and lead productive lives.

The amputees who shared their stories in this book were all ordinary people leading their respectively ordinary lives. Accidents, progressive diseases, and congenital disabilities resulted in the loss of one or multiple limbs for each of them.

Larry, our 80-year-old, bilateral amputee still walks, gardens, and cherishes his time with his grandchildren. Carol, takes care of all her own activities independently, even with the loss of all her limbs. She walks daily and loves her retirement years socializing and spending time with her family. Ray walks his dog and attends church and is passionate that he is not ready to give up although he has been given multiple death diagnoses. Carlos took his amputation in stride starting a support group and is active as a peer counselor. Jon continues to work for the utility company, plays with his family, and leads a very active life.

Megan has married, and she and her husband just had their first child. She works full time and is very busy balancing her family life and work life—and is no longer concerned about her appearance! Jake started farming in New Zealand and has incorporated all of his upper and lower prosthetics into his daily chores. He takes each challenge with positivity and creativity. Life after limb loss is an individual journey for all amputees and their families. You are never alone. You have peers, loved ones, and a medical team available throughout your journey to help you. By definition, a hero is a person who is brave, admired for their courage and outstanding achievements, and is regarded as a role model. All amputees are heroes as they strive for their best selves—their futures bright with a life well lived just around the corner.

Acknowledgements

The biggest thank you possible to my business partner, writing coach, and mentor, Sean Sumner PT. This book was his idea, and his constant encouragement kept me on a forward course. Writing a book never entered my consciousness until he suggested I take this great challenge on. Seeing it through to fruition is beyond anything I thought possible.

Thank you to all the featured amputees: Larry, Carol, Carlos, Megan, Jon, and Jake who were each an inspiration to me and were gracious in allowing me to share their personal stories.

A special thank you to all the prosthetists that have taught me so much and have helped me gain the skills in prosthetics. Specifically, thank you to Bryan Hayes, CPO, Dave Scurti, CPO, and Mike Shower, CPO who for over the past 20 years have worked with me and make up such a special team.

And to Dr. Chris Shin, whose knowledge, skill, and teaching continue to help me grow both professionally and personally. I am a better clinician and person because of your support and friendship.

Made in the USA
San Bernardino, CA
24 February 2019